Myths & Facts

around

Diet & Exercise

AF776204

Myths & Facts

around

Diet & Exercise

Prashant Surana

MOONLIGHT BOOKS

Myths & Facts around Diet & Exercise

FIRST EDITION: 2023

ISBN PB: 978-93-92756-74-0
ISBN EBOOK: 978-93-92756-69-6

Copyright © *Prashant Surana*

Published by
MOONLIGHT BOOKS
20 Ekjot Apartment, Pitampura, Delhi - 110034
Email : moonlightbooks2016@gmail.com
www.moonlightbooks.in

All rights reserved. No part of this book may be used or reproduced in any manner whatsoever, including Internet usage, without permission from the publisher, except in the case of brief quotations embodied in critical articles and reviews.

Designed by Omnis Communications, India

Printed by Replika Press Pvt. Ltd., India

"Health is the greatest gift,

contentment the greatest wealth,

faithfulness the best relationship."

–Buddha

Preface

Satyameva Jayate (truth alone triumphs).

Truth is a kind of information, and so is untruth. These days, in the age of internet and smartphones, we feel strangely empowered – we have the power to get all the information we seek, instantly, at the swipe of a finger, at the command of our voice...

However, every bit of information is not necessarily a truth. It could be a fact, a distorted factoid or downright 'fake news'. When all these are served mixed up on the same platform, how are you to tell what is true and what is not?

Even the latest rage, the Artificial Intelligence systems like ChatGPT cannot come to your rescue because these are trained on the same 'mixture' that is already available on the internet, and the latest stuff is not even included in the free version. That is one reason why AI cannot replace humans entirely – machines may become intelligent but only human beings can attain wisdom.

And then there is the so called 'conventional wisdom' – passed on down the generations, along cultural lines and ethnic lineages. The test of modern scientific inquiry routinely shows that some of these are indeed 'wisdom', but the rest are just 'conventional'. How would you know the difference?

Due to increased media exposure and heightened self-consciousness towards looking good, 'diet & exercise' has now become the hottest subject for content consumption. Most of this happens on social media, which is the greatest myth-multiplier in the history of humankind. Anything presented in an interesting or shocking manner goes viral, and the recipients mostly do not fact-check the claims being made, because either they don't have the temperament to challenge it or don't have the technical background for it. All this has given birth to a new beast called 'digital disinformation'.

"While misinformation refers to the accidental spread of inaccurate information, disinformation is not only inaccurate, but intends to deceive and is spread in order to do serious harm" (United Nations).

Many a times we continue to believe in something because we want to believe in it, because it makes us feel good about what we already think or do. At times we get influenced by the physical appearance of the person making the claim – someone with a great body is assumed to be an expert on exercise and someone doing yoga poses nicely is assumed to be a yoga expert - which may not be the case, just as being a great cook is not the same as being an expert on nutrition!

As the saying in Hindi goes: *pehla sukh, nirogi kaya* – the first order of happiness is to have a healthy body. It's an irony that we are mostly ill-informed about the very issues that affect our health the most: what to eat... how to exercise... Therefore, this book is an effort to address the myths around diet, exercise and health that we routinely come across, either on social media or in casual conversations. As far as possible, I have tried to explain the underlying scientific facts while leaving out the technical jargon, to make it an easy read irrespective of a reader's background.

Even if you are not seriously into dieting or exercising, you will be surprised to note that so many of our beliefs, routine activities or choices that we make on daily basis are on the not-so-healthy side, and to that extent, everyone can expect to get some benefit out of this curated collection of myths and facts.

Let us get vaccinated against the fake news virus!

--Prashant Surana

Contents

1.

Body is like a machine...

Nope!

We tend to think of our body as a machine. Modern healthcare practice, compartmentalised into various specialists, also promotes this concept, because just like complex machines, the body is supposed to consist of various specialised parts that work together to keep us alive and functional.

It was none other than the great Leonardo da Vinci (of Mona Lisa fame) who pioneered this attitude by comparing our muscles and bones to a system of ropes, levers and pulleys.

There is a fundamental flaw in this kind of thinking. Machines are designed for predictable output or behaviour. If you change one variable, while keeping other variables constant, the output or behaviour changes proportionately. For example, if you press the accelerator of your car harder, it speeds up in a predictable manner, every time. When you apply brakes, it comes to a stop obediently.

Our bodies, in contrast, are the result of millions of years of evolution – which essentially is a hit and trial process. Any functionality that helped our survival and reproduction in the past has been retained, and the same kicks in as soon as similar circumstances arise, whether we want it or not, whether we like it or not.

Take a look at these examples:

1. Calorie-rich food was scarce for our hunter-gatherer ancestors. Those who found such food very appealing and gorged on it, were better nourished and hence more capable of surviving and reproducing, therefore had more surviving kids who in turn again had more surviving kids. Those with this trait thus soon outnumbered others and became dominant. This is how evolution works.

2. Individuals who can store fat quickly when food is abundant and burn this fat slowly when they go hungry, had a survival advantage in the event of a famine – something the human population faced frequently until recent history. As a result, this trait is now in the genes of most of us. It makes us put on weight quickly and makes it pretty hard to lose it - as anyone struggling to lose weight will readily testify. Our bodies evolved not to prevent obesity, but to prevent us from dying of starvation, which was a real and frequent possibility until the modern times.

3. Among our ancestors, those who were not afraid of snakes, were more likely to have been bitten by snakes,

died young and got removed from the gene pool. The rest, who were afraid, survived and reproduced, and hence now the fear of snakes is a wide-spread human tendency.

4. Those who could not feel pain, died young because of recklessness and were removed from the gene pool. Those who felt pain, took better care of their bodies, avoided danger and thus survived and multiplied. Thus, sense and fear of pain is now permanently encoded in the genes of almost all the creatures.

5. The last 2 examples show how unpleasant sensations like fear, pain, anxiety etc. confer protective advantages and become entrenched during evolution. The evolutionary processes therefore work for preserving and multiplying life itself, not for ensuring our happiness or pleasures.

As a result of this evolutionary programming, our bodies try to resist change. If you change one variable, the body will adjust other variables and try to keep the output constant! In fact, keeping certain variables within a set of vital ranges is the main function of many of our body's systems, because that's what keeps us alive!

On the contrary, we expect the body to behave predictably like a machine. We make a small change in our lifestyle and expect immediate and lasting results from it. When we start dieting or exercise, we expect that our weight will start going down and will continue to go down as long as we continue to diet/exercise. We aggressively avoid sugar and fat to lose weight and get frustrated when nothing happens. We go on crash diets to get slim and then expect to remain that way forever. Some of us go to great lengths to look like models and film stars without an awareness of the unwanted negative effects it can have on the body and mind.

Going forward, as we dive deeper into many such issues, do keep this fact at the back of your mind – body is not a machine, it is a self-organising system that has evolved over millions of years, and it tries to resist change. Whatever changes you attempt to bring to it, do not expect immediate results.

It also works the other way round – just as good things do not show immediate positive results, bad things may not show immediate negative results. As usual, our body tries to compensate and keep going, until it no longer can. This give us a false sense of 'all is well' and we just keep going as usual.

For example, if something is damaging the kidneys, we will not know until 80% of the kidneys are gone, because only then you start feeling the symptoms. Ditto for the liver. Smoking seems harmless at the moment, but the negative effects accumulate over decades and eventually diseases ensue. Few extra calories consumed on a daily basis can raise your weight by a few imperceptible grams per day, which keep adding up and become tens of kilograms over the years.

It is because of these adaptive and compensatory mechanisms that our body does not behave according to what our common sense or intuition would predict. As you might have heard doctors saying, in medical science 2+2 is not always equal to 4...!

2.

Prefer light / low fat food...

Don't!

A common misconception most of us have is that whatever we eat gets deposited in the body. So, if we eat fat, it will make us fat. If we eat heavy (heavy to digest) food, it will make us heavy. Therefore, many of us develop a preference for light and easy to digest food. Particularly those who are dieting or otherwise trying to lose weight or just trying to maintain a healthy lifestyle.

Please note: our body is an active bio-chemical factory, not a passive pipeline attached to storage facilities. Whatever we eat, gets shredded down to the basic molecules, which are then recombined as per the needs of various body tissues.

The body can convert everything into calories when required, and conversely excess calories consumed in any form can be converted to fat and stored.

Therefore, when you are dieting, you need to consume overall less calories than you burn in 24 hours. Cutting out fat alone (or for that matter any particular type of food) does not work.

On the contrary, leaving out fat from your diet may cause deficiency of fat-soluble vitamins and other fat-soluble nutrients, such as (not a complete list, there are many more)...

- Vitamin A – necessary for health of eyes, skin and immunity.
- Vitamin D – necessary for absorbing calcium from food, also prevents many chronic diseases
- Vitamin E – necessary to maintain the health of all cell membranes.
- Vitamin K – involved in clotting of blood in case of injury, wound healing, bone and lung health
- Omega 3 fatty acids – keep inflammation in check, prevent many chronic diseases

What is mostly stored as fat in the body then? See the following graph:

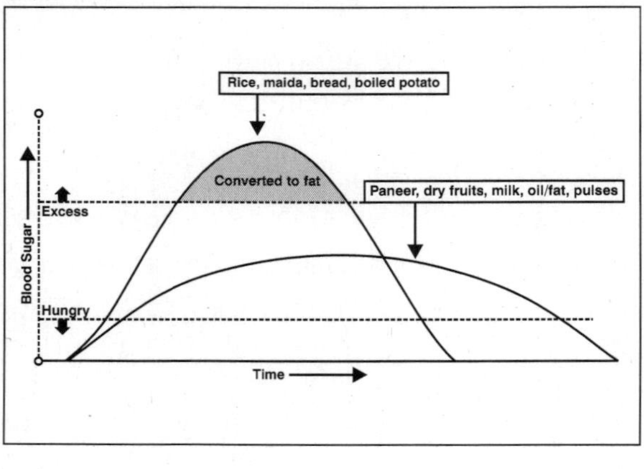

Whenever you eat, all that can be broken down to sugar (glucose) by the digestive system, gets converted to sugar and is absorbed into the blood circulation along with other nutrients. This glucose is the basic and essential fuel that our cells need to survive and function, and therefore the body tries to maintain a certain level of it in the blood. If the level goes down, you feel hungry. If the level goes up beyond a certain level, the excess glucose is converted to fat and stored. That is where most of the fat piling up in our body actually comes from, not from the fat that you eat!

When you eat 'easy to digest' stuff that can be quickly converted to glucose, such as sugar, rice, bread and biscuits etc. made of refined flour (*maida*), boiled potato or other such starchy foodstuff, the blood sugar level quicky rises and a part of it is converted to fat as shown. Since that part is now removed from the blood, the blood sugar level quickly drops (the rest being used up by the body as fuel). This makes you feel hungry soon, and if you eat the same kind of stuff again, this cycle keeps repeating and with each cycle some fat gets deposited in your body.

Take a look at the following graph... What is most likely to be converted to fat? What will make you feel hungry sooner?

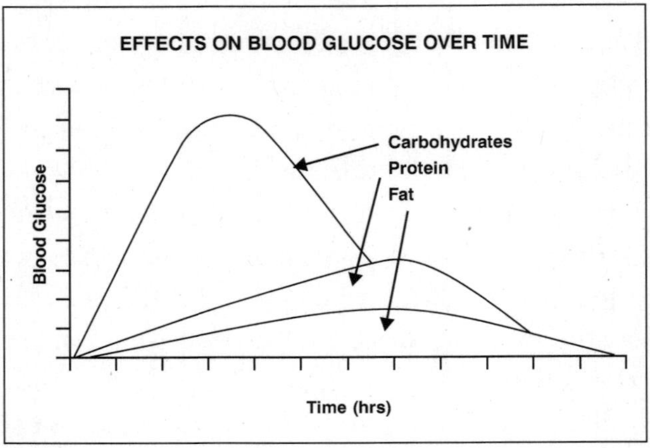

Does that mean we should exclude carbohydrates (starchy foods) completely? If we do, the body will have to get all the glucose it needs by breaking down fats and proteins, which comes with its own repertoire of toxic by-products and digestive discomforts. Not a good idea. In general, cutting out any foodstuff entirely is a bad idea because each comes as a package deal – a collection of many different nutrients. When you give up something entirely then you miss this entire package. Instead, try to have more variety in your food so that you get a wide variety of nutrients. Small quantity, more variety – that's the way to go.

All you need to do is to reduce, as much as you practically can, the quantity of the easy to digest types – sugary liquids, breads, biscuits, other refined flour items, boiled rice, boiled potato, cornflakes, other boiled starchy stuff such as *sabudana* (sago), *idli*, *appam* etc.

The boiling of starch merits particular mention. When you boil starchy stuff like potato, it's not just boiling – the boiling water actually has a chemical reaction with the starch (called hydrolysis), which breaks it down and makes it particularly easy to digest.

In case of potato the contrast is particularly stark. When you boil it, many water-soluble nutrients are lost in the water that you just throw away. The boiled (hydrolysed) starch becomes easily digestible and shoots up your blood sugar level when you eat it. On the contrary, baked potatoes are healthy because no nutrients are lost, and the starch (just heated and cooled but not hydrolysed) becomes more complex and therefore gets digested slowly. The humble potato can go from healthy to unhealthy depending on how you cook!

The Europeans conquered the world while eating baked potatoes on their ships, on the other hand India has become the diabetes capital of the world while eating boiled potatoes in every conceivable form!

Steamed south Indian staples like *idli* and *appam* are the crowning glory of the easy to digest variety! These are considered very healthy by most of us, but just consider this: these are fermented and then steamed. Fermentation already half-digests the starch in it and then you steam it... No wonder you feel hungry shortly after such a meal.

Add to this boiled rice, and it becomes easy to understand why a recent National Family Health Survey found South Indians to be more obese than the national average.

At this juncture many of you might be wondering about fruits... What about the sugar in fruits? Well, fruits contain sugar in the form of fructose mainly, which our liver has to convert to glucose. This takes some time and therefore the blood sugar level does not rise immediately after eating. Also, fruits have lots of fibre which slow down the absorption process – this is also the reason why fruits are alright, but fruit juices are not so healthy. See the graph below, which shows blood sugar profile of an apple compared with equal amount of glucose powder:

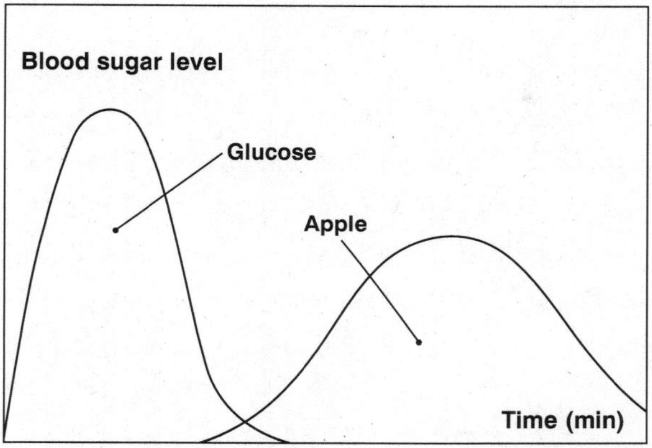

It's not just what you eat, what you do after eating also has an impact on your blood sugar levels and therefore on fat accumulation. If you go to sleep after a meal, blood sugar levels rise higher and if you are active after the meal the blood sugar levels are lower. Consider the graph below*:

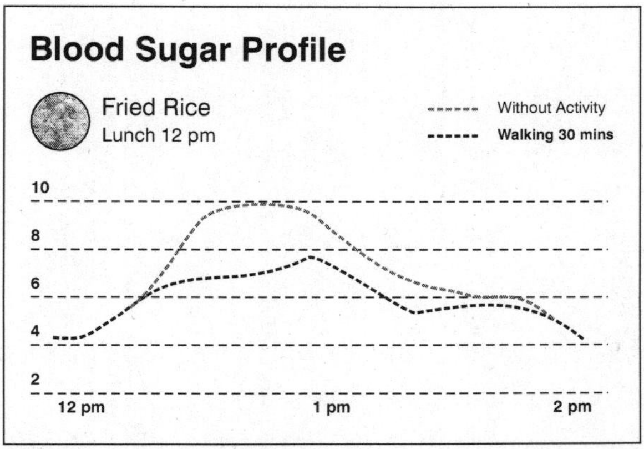

*Please Note: Fried rice is not actually fried; it is just boiled rice with some oil added.

In addition to what you eat and what you do after eating, another important factor is your age. Youngsters have faster metabolisms, so their bodies use up the blood sugar quickly, and therefore the blood sugar does not go high enough to convert to fat and also comes down quickly. This is the reason teenagers usually are hungry all the

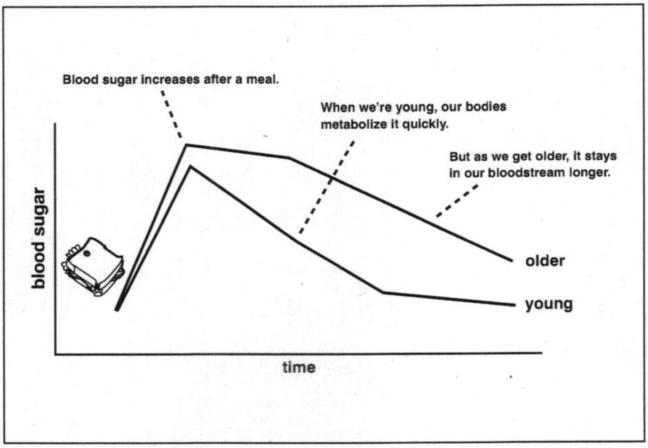

time, eat all kinds of junk yet don't gain weight (mostly... though teenage obesity is also on the rise these days). As we get older, metabolism slows down, and blood sugar goes higher even as we are eating the same food in the same quantity.

This is the reason why we start gaining weight as move towards our 30s and if we don't change our lifestyle and food habits, we continue on that upward trajectory. Females have lower metabolic rate than males, so they are at greater risk of gaining weight with increasing age. Various surveys also consistently report higher rates of obesity in women than in men.

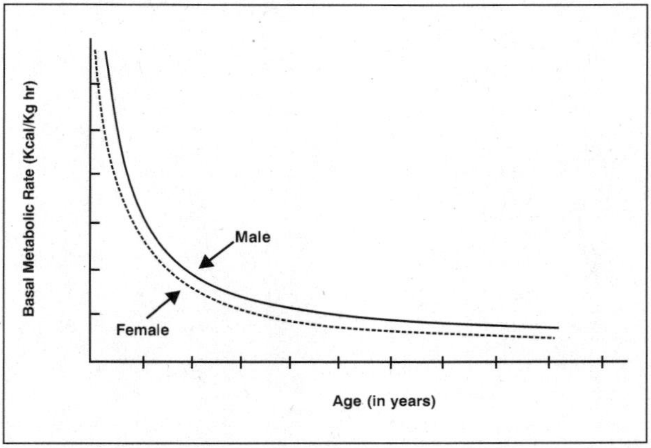

Our metabolic rate (the total calories we burn in 24 hours) continues to decrease with age, but our diet gets fixed sometime around 20 years of age. At that age the diet was alright, but as you get older this diet starts to give you extra calories because your metabolic rate is falling. These extra calories pile up as fat in your body.

What's the way out...? The obvious answer: reduce your calorie intake as you age. At least eat less of the easy to digest category that pushes up your blood sugar rapidly. You can add more fibre in your diet to slow down the rate of absorption – you can do this by adding fibre rich grains such as millets to the wheat flour. Consume whole fruits instead of juices.

The not so obvious answer: increase your muscle mass! See this graph below:

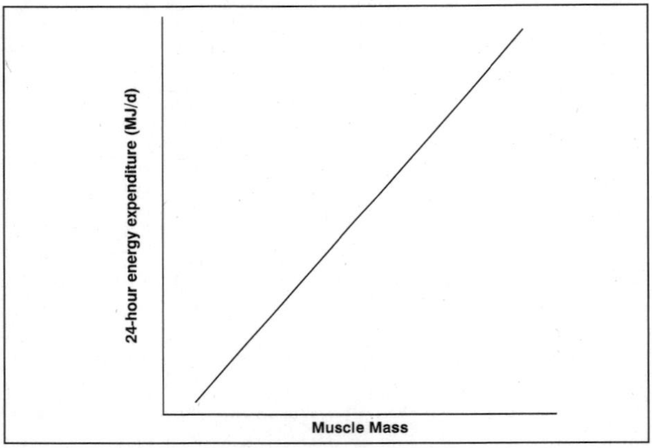

The bigger the muscles you have on your body, the more calories you burn over 24 hours, even if you don't use them. It's like the engine of a truck consuming more fuel than a car even while idling on a red light.

Regular weights training + sufficient proteins in the diet can significantly increase and maintain your muscle mass. Yoga also provides modest muscle mass improvement.

Both of these also have other beneficial effects, including slow aging, increased lifespan, lower risk of chronic diseases etc. that we will discuss further down this book.

The male hormones in men make it easier for them to gain and maintain significant muscle mass, not so with women. So, the ladies have to be more careful with their diet. On the other hand, extra fat troubles men more than women, as the risk of fat related chronic diseases like high BP, diabetes, heart disease etc. is much higher in men than in women. Nature's balancing act, I guess...!

3.

Fat = Cholesterol = Problem...

Not Exactly!

In the last chapter, when we said that consuming fat is in fact necessary and healthy in moderation, this question must have popped in your mind: what about cholesterol?

It is common knowledge these days that fat consumption raises cholesterol levels – which gets deposited in the coronary arteries and causes heart disease, technically known as cardiovascular disease (CVD).

As a result, many companies selling cooking oils etc. tout their low cholesterol level or cholesterol lowering properties. Many of us try to avoid dairy fats (milk, curd, cheese, butter, *ghee*) because these are supposed to be high in cholesterol.

Is cholesterol really the villain?

Cholesterol is an essential ingredient for life. Food is not the only source as every animal and human cell is capable of manufacturing its own cholesterol, but this goes up and down depending on how much we get from food - thus, the body automatically maintains the required levels. And therefore, only food from animal source contains cholesterol.

Consider this:

- Our cell membranes are 30% cholesterol.
- It is essential for the health of our nervous system.
- It is the raw material for synthesis of Vitamin D and many hormones including sex hormones.
- It is a major component of our skin and is responsible for making it waterproof.

Also consider this: everyone having high cholesterol levels does not have heart disease. And everyone having heart disease does not necessarily have high cholesterol!

So obviously cholesterol is not the only villain... There is something else going on here. This 'something else' is inflammation.

Inflammation is body's response that supplies healing and infection-fighting material to an injured tissue. So, in the short term, it is a good thing because it has a healing or repairing effect. But sustained low level inflammation can irritate the inner lining of the blood vessels, particularly those supplying blood to the heart (coronary arteries). Circulating cholesterol in the blood can then stick to this irritated lining and gradually become a plaque (a pad like build up). The plaque can itself block the artery or it can loosen/burst and trigger formation of blood clot. This blood clot can block the coronary artery leading to a heart attack or it can block an artery in the brain causing a srtoke.

The sustained low-level inflammation, which starts this cascade of damning events in the first place, occurs when something is damaging body tissues slowly and continuously over a period of time, such as smoking, pollution, high blood sugar, high blood pressure, stress etc. Accumulated fat also promotes inflammation in the body. Increasing age also increases inflammation due to accumulated cellular defects.

How can we reduce this kind of inflammation?

Some answers are obvious – quit smoking, change diet as discussed in previous chapter to reduce blood sugar, get rid of excess body fat, manage stress, etc.

The not so obvious answer: exercise. Physical exercise can reduce inflammation through various mechanisms:

- It makes heavy energy demand on the body, so our body withdraws energy being spent in unnecessary processes, inflammation being one of them.
- It helps reduce blood sugar levels.
- Improves blood circulation – this makes oxygen and nutrients move more efficiently to repair the damaged tissues and thus resolves the inflammation faster.
- Exercise is known to reduce stress levels.

- Not just heart disease, a recent study shows that vigorous physical activity of as much 5 minutes per day can cut risk of cancer by 20%.

Therefore, the real villain of this story is not cholesterol, but inflammation. And the real hero that can defeat this villain, is exercise.

However, those who have been prescribed medication to lower cholesterol because they already have CVD or are at high risk, must continue to take their medicines. These meds reduce cholesterol and also inflammation to some extent. Do not go against medical advice.

Coming back to the question of fats. Now that we know cholesterol alone is not the issue, there are also other reasons why dairy fats or milk fats are not as bad as most of us believe. There are recent studies that show that these actually have a protective effect on the heart when consumed in moderation, as compared to other types of fats.

The protective effect of milk fats may be attributed to the following reasons:

- The milk fat is not a single substance, these are complex natural mixtures, and the composition possibly has a beneficial effect on the heart.
- As already discussed, these contain many fat-soluble vitamins, proteins and other such nutrients

which have a positive effect on the overall health, thus indirectly promoting heart health.

- These fats make you feel full and satisfied much faster, thus some of us may end up consuming less calories and other unhealthy foods, which in turn helps manage weight and heart disease risk.
- The fermented milk products like curd, buttermilk, yoghurt and cheese also promote beneficial gut bacteria, which reduce inflammation.
- Milk is rich in calcium and also provides some amount of Vitamin D, both necessary for bone health.

Another food that has a similar protective effect: Nuts, also known as dry fruits (almonds, cashews, pistachios, walnuts, pekans, melon seeds, sunflower seeds, pumpkin seeds, peanuts etc.)

Nuts have beneficial fats and fat-soluble nutrients, fibre, protein, antioxidants, minerals etc. and zero cholesterol! But just as with everything else in life, enjoy in moderation, because nuts also pack quite a punch in calories.

Many food products are marketed as 'non-dairy' and 'low cholesterol' to encash the popular psyche against dairy (milk) fat and cholesterol. Many of these products use hydrogenated vegetable oils as a replacement – which are cholesterol free but may actually harm the heart-health as per recent studies, and also do not contain all those nutrients as in natural milk fat.

Any discussion on fats would be incomplete without mentioning ice cream. This universally popular treat is around 10 to 20 percent fat by weight. A lot of this weight is water; hence 100 gm ice cream contains around 200 calories - which is not much, considering 100 gm *gulab jamun* contains 700 calories.

In India, ice creams are commercially available under two labels as per government regulations. Those labelled as 'ice cream' contain milk fat, while those labelled as 'frozen dessert' contain hydrogenated vegetable oils with or without milk components. Just for your information...!

4.

Dieting = Fasting...

Not True!

As discussed in earlier chapters, we can change our diet in such a way that the part that is converted to fat is minimised. This, coupled with increased muscle mass to burn more calories overall, is the optimal strategy to lose weight or maintain healthy weight and maintain overall health.

However, there are many who believe that fasting is the way to lose weight, which means going hungry frequently or regularly skipping a meal or eating very little in each meal, because of the belief that our weight is all about how much food we consume. While this sounds very intuitive, it can actually defeat the very objective you are trying to achieve, because of the negative effects it can have on the body and mind.

Here are various negative effects of fasting for weight loss:

A hungry body learns to conserve calories. Frequent or extended fasting makes the body slow down its metabolism. Remember the first chapter – the body tries to compensate because its first priority is to survive. So, when less calories are available routinely, it slows down its activities to burn less calories. Now when you resume your regular eating schedule, your slowed down metabolism will burn less calories and store more of it as fat. No wonder many who go fasting to lose weight - regain more weight than they had lost initially when they start eating normally again.

A hungry body converts everything to calories. When you try to burn fat rapidly by extended or frequent fasting, it is not just fat that is consumed in the process, but also muscles. When you lose muscle mass, your metabolic rate goes down and you burn less calories even at rest. We already discussed how increased muscle mass makes you burn more calories – this is just the opposite of that. Decreasing muscle mass also makes you physically weak and frail. In extreme cases, the body may shut down the reproductive system (not necessary for survival) to conserve calories, resulting in infertility.

A hungry body is a malnourished body.
Prolonged/frequent fasting can reduce the overall intake of essential nutrients and can therefore cause various kinds of deficiencies. This can result in other health issues and decreased energy levels. One important consequence is bone loss or weakening of bones – nutritional and hormonal factors come together to cause bone loss during

fasting. Weak muscles and weak bones can combine to increase the incidence of falls and fractures.

A hungry body is a dull body. Due to factors described above, one can feel lethargy, tiredness and low energy due to fasting. Your blood sugar levels may drop, which can lead to fatigue and difficulty in concentrating. You brain uses up 20% of the calories you consume – when calories are in short supply, the supply to the brain is also restricted, impacting its performance. Not at all good for students, intellectuals or problem solvers.

A hungry body has a disturbed mind. All the issues discussed above can converge to disturb the mind and lead to disorders like binge eating, irritability, anger, anxiety, mood swings, impaired cognition and lower productivity.

There is one more serious consequence of prolonged/frequent fasting, which may not happen to everyone, but the risk is always present. Our gallbladder is a small pouch on the side of the liver. It receives bile from the liver and secretes it into the intestine for fat digestion. When food reaches the stomach, it releases a hormone that causes the muscles around the gallbladder to contract and release the bile. When you don't eat, this hormone is not released and the bile remains in the gallbladder, where it can become very concentrated over time and turn into stones. If one is also losing weight rapidly as result of this fasting, then flow of bile from the liver is also increased due to increased fat metabolism. So, more inflow and less outflow – further increases the risk of gallbladder stones.

In the recent past, the concept of 'Autophagy' has gained a lot of currency on the internet and social media. It implies the recycling of cellular waste within a living cell. In response to starvation or nutrient restriction the cell digests unwanted or waste components into raw material which are then used for the synthesis of components that are essential for survival. This recycling process is supposed to repair or rejuvenate the cells and therefore slow down aging, improve health and prevent chronic diseases. This is autophagy (literal meaning: eating oneself).

All that is very well and good, but there are a few misconceptions that need to be addressed:

- Fasting is the only way to induce autophagy: No, physical exercise also induces autophagy. Nutrient scarcity can be created either by decreasing the supply (fasting) or by increasing the demand (exercise). In fact, this is supposed to be one of the reasons why exercise reduces inflammation and slows down aging.
- Prolonged/frequent fasting is required to get full benefit of autophagy (or the more the merrier):

No, our cells are not so choke-a-block with waste products that they will continue to do autophagy as long as you are fasting. Occasional / short duration fasting, or exercise is enough to trigger autophagy.

- Given the negative side effects of fasting and positive effects of exercise, it should be clear that exercise would be a much better way to induce autophagy, if at all.

Another social media darling of recent vintage is 'Intermittent Fasting'. It is not fasting in the true sense of the word, it should actually be called 'time restricted eating', because you don't go hungry for long periods, and you don't significantly restrict your calorie intake. Of course, if one is in the habit of eating all the time, then the time restriction will also result in calorie restriction, but that would be a healthy restriction and will cause a healthy fat/weight loss.

There are various popular patterns, like eating over 8 hours and going hungry for 16 hours (of which 8 hours should be sleep), having an early dinner or not eating after sunset (long practised in Jainism out of religious beliefs), eating on alternate days (more extreme, not recommended) and the 5:2 plan –eating 5 days a week normally and then eating one meal a day on weekends.

Part of the benefit of this regimented lifestyle comes from the discipline itself – a disciplined lifestyle is a healthy one. A lot of junk calories are consumed by us during snacking – and intermittent fasting effectively limits snacking. This itself can result is weight loss or help maintain healthy weight.

This kind of time restriction can also induce autophagy with all its consequent benefits. It also provides much needed rest to our digestive and metabolic systems, improving their function and thus overall health.

One more indirect benefit is that you don't go to bed soon after dinner, which, if you recall chapter 2, keeps your post-dinner blood sugar levels on the healthy side and helps prevent conversion to fat. This is something you can do even without calling it intermittent fasting. Take your pick...!

5.

Dieting is complicated...

If you follow social media!

Dieting is the name of the conscious efforts that you make to reduce your weight and body fat. All it means is to consume less calories than you typically burn in 24 hours. This can be achieved simply by reducing the portion size of your regular meals, snacks etc. Just remove 20-30% of your regular quantity and put it aside or give it to someone else. This is a natural, non-shocking way of nudging the body towards using more of the stored calories. It is all about consuming less, not about consuming some special food. Just continue with your usual food and reduce or avoid the easy to digest types, if at all.

The culinary culture or food habits of each culture are derived from their natural environment – and passed along through social learning. Before global supply chains started making everything available everywhere, people ate what was locally available and learned to make the best of it. If their food habits were a good fit with the environment, the population thrived – so if your community has survived and multiplied, then your ancestral grandmas and aunties must have been doing something right in their kitchens; those traditional foods and diets should not be given up just like that, in the name of special diets for weight loss.

Another important concept to understand is that your weight is a function of your lifestyle. Whatever changes you are making to lose weight, will have to be maintained to keep that weight. If you go back to the old lifestyle, you will go back to the old weight. That is because when you lose weight, the calories you burn over 24 hours also goes down (the fat you have lost was also burning some calories). Once your calorie intake reaches an equilibrium with your calorie expenditure, your weight becomes constant, and you have to maintain this equilibrium to maintain this weight. If you increase your calorie intake now by going back to the old habits, your weight starts rising again. When this happens, your 24-hour calorie expenditure also increases, until you reach a new equilibrium where your intake balances your expenditure. This is you new weight. This is what we call 'yoyo dieting' – wherein people keep losing and gaining weight in cycles of dieting and normal eating.

Therefore, when you switch to a special diet to lose weight, be mindful that if you want your weight loss to be permanent, you will have to maintain yourself on this diet for the rest of your life. If you cannot visualise yourself on that diet for the rest of your life, then just apply portion control on your traditional food.

Today, on the internet and social media you can find a cacophony of various dieting strategies claiming various health benefits and physical results. It can sound rather complicated with all the jargon and buzzwords being thrown around.

Here, just for the sake of information and to demystify the jargon, is a summary of the popular diets and their pros and cons:

Mediterranean Diet:

Pros: Emphasis on fruits, vegetables, whole grains, and healthy fats (olive oil, nuts, seeds), which may reduce the risk of heart disease and other chronic diseases.

Cons: High fat and calorie content, portion control is essential to avoid weight gain.

Ketogenic Diet / Atkins Diet / Low-carb Diet:

Pros: Very low or zero carbs, can lead to rapid weight loss due to burning of fat for fuel (ketosis). Helps control blood sugar levels and may benefit people with epilepsy or certain neurological disorders.

Cons: Unnatural, causes side effects and digestive discomforts. Difficult to maintain long term.

Paleo Diet:

Pros: Focuses on whole foods, meats without fats, fruits, vegetables, nuts and seeds. No processed foods, refined sugars, and grains (all easy to digest), which may help with weight loss and inflammation reduction.

Cons: Certain food groups are absent (like milk, grains and legumes or pulses), which may lead to deficiencies. Not enough scientific evidence on long-term health benefits.

These special diets are designed with a focus on the calories and on the macronutrients like proteins, carbs, fats etc. But our diet is not just energy and macronutrients; there are hundreds of micronutrients that we need in minute quantities. We get these by including more variety in our diet. Restricting the diet to a few foodstuffs that are repeated everyday may sound more disciplined, but it actually deprives the body from receiving the full range of micronutrients and is therefore not healthy in the long run.

The traditional Indian cuisine is so unique and complex in its composition that it is difficult to fit it in these moulds of special diets. The possible tweaks you can apply without causing wholesale upheaval in the Indian kitchen are as follows:

- Add high fibre grains like millets to wheat while making flour for chapattis etc.
- Minimise stuff made of refined flour (*maida*) and try to use less finely milled flour.
- Eat more of seeds/pulses/legumes/vegetables and less of fermented/boiled starches (bread, rice, potato, *naan*, *kulcha*, *idli*, *appam* etc.).
- Minimise the amount of oil used in seasoning (*tadka/chhonk*) of the dishes.
- Include milk/milk products, curd and nuts in moderation.

Bon appétit...!

6.

Obese people are careless...

No, it may be a genetic burden!

Becoming overweight or obese or fat is usually assumed to be the person's own fault. We tend to take it for granted that such a person is careless about eating, is given to overeating or is a glutton.

This may actually be true in a few cases, but mostly their genes should get the blame rather than their mouths.

The modern lifestyle can further add fuel this fire that is already burning bright due to genetic tendencies. Genetic factors working together with food and lifestyle choices make a person prone to gaining weight and storing fat. If your genes try to make you fat but your choices are correct, then maybe you will end up slightly overweight. But if with the same genes you make poor choices then you can become morbidly obese. Similarly, two people eating the same food can end up with different body weights depending on their genes.

There is a strong correlation between 'Frame Size' and weight gain. Frame size refers to the width of our skeletal frame. Larger frame size means a wider body. People with larger frames gain weight easily.

Frame size is measured by wrist circumference, which is measured by measuring the circumference of the wrist around the same point where we can check our pulse. The average male wrist circumference is 6.9 inches and that of female is 6 inches. Anyone having significantly larger wrist circumference than these averages has a large frame size. Generally, 5.5 - 6.5 inches are considered a small wrist, 6.5 - 7 inches a medium wrist and 7+ inches a large wrist, and thereby the corresponding frame size.

People with large frame sizes have larger stomachs and more powerful digestive systems. They digest food faster, leading to higher blood sugar levels and faster drop in blood sugar levels because a part of it is converted to fat. This makes them store more fat and also makes them feel hungry much faster. The increased hunger makes them eat more the next time or to snack in between meals. All these factors combine to make them gain weight.

Therefore, it is not surprising that larger wrist circumference has a high correlation with the incidence of high BP, heart disease and diabetes.

People with smaller frame sizes on the other hand find it difficult to gain weight, at least until the middle age. Most of the so-called fashion models have small frames, helping them stay slim and stave off weight gain. But the flip side is that people with small frames have lower muscle mass and low bone density.

Those with larger frames can add muscle mass easily if/when they do physical exercise like weights training. This is their best solution to manage their weight as it increases the metabolic rate (larger muscles burn more calories even at rest) and also brings a host of other benefits such as reduced inflammation, slower aging and lesser risk of various chronic diseases.

That does not mean weights training is useless for those with smaller frame sizes. For them, weights training can correct their low muscle mass and low bone density and improve stamina, though they will not gain huge muscles like those with larger frames.

Awareness of this concept of frame sizes therefore also helps maintain realistic expectations from one's body. If one wants a body like Arnold Schwarzenegger, ones should first have his wrist circumference of 7.5 inches. What's yours...?

7.

Obesity is all about eating wrong…

No, there is a lot more to it!

The previous chapter might have made you think that due to frame size or whatever reason, some people just overeat or eat the wrong kind of food and become obese. But it's not that simple. The reality is a bit more complex. While frame size is a broad concept applicable to all of us, there are other factors at play as well – genetic as well as environmental.

Here are the different reasons why people gain weight, apart from having a large frame size or eating the wrong types of food:

1. Fast Digestion: Some individuals may have fast digestions in spite having a normal or small frame size. Their stomach gets empty faster, the blood sugar rises rapidly – a part of which is converted to fat, and then they are hungry again shortly after eating. Thus, they eat more frequently, get more of

their calories converted to fat and therefore become obese over a period of time due to this multiplier effect. This could also happen if one has a larger than normal stomach size.

2. Late Satiety: The brain of such people does not recognise or responds to the signals that stomach is full, or responds with a delay. This makes them continue to feel hungry even when technically they have eaten enough. Thus, they end up consuming more calories than they need. These extra calories consumed on a regular basis makes them obese.

3. Tardy Metabolism: Some of us may have slow metabolism in our genes. Such individuals burn comparatively lesser calories in 24 hours, and the unused extra calories get accumulated as fat in the body. They have low energy levels and find it difficult to engage in physical activity. They gain weight even as they are eating right.

4. Emotional Cravings: It is a well-known fact that eating high calorie food makes us feel good. We are naturally programmed to feel rewarded when we eat certain stuff (sweet, delicious, high calorie) because of the ancient evolutionary advantages that came with it. Therefore, it is not surprising that negative emotions like low self-esteem, feelings of

inadequacy, anxiety and depression etc. can trigger cravings for such food, due to the activation of reward seeking circuits in the brain. Such behaviour over a period of time can result in weight gain. Research shows that chronic stress, plus a high-calorie diet, can drive more and more food intake as well as a preference for sweet, delicious food, thereby promoting weight gain and obesity. This highlights that a healthy diet is even more crucial during times of stress.

5. Cultural Strings: Some families traditionally eat food that is high in calories with excessive fat content (oil/butter/*ghee*) or a large proportion of 'easy to digest' starchy stuff. Kids raised in such households have no option but to eat it and they grow up to love such food as they develop a taste for it over time – thus perpetuating the tradition. Some cultures traditionally consume larger portions and find it difficult to control portion sizes when advised to.

6. Anxious Parents: Some over-anxious parents tend to force-feed their kids, making them habitual over-eaters for the rest of their lives. These parents are overly scared of kids going hungry or not eating enough and misjudge the portion size that should be allocated for kids compared to grown-ups. Kids have smaller stomachs so need smaller portions but tend

to eat more frequently due to their faster metabolism. Overeating causes the stomach to expand beyond its normal size to adjust to the large amount of food, as a result these kids may grow up to have stomachs larger than what is dictated by their frame sizes, thus turning them into the category 1 above.

Having seen the various reasons why people gain weight or become obese in the modern society, let us also discuss the solutions the modern society offers in order to solve this problem, apart from the obvious 'eat less - eat right – exercise more' kind of advisory one gets showered with.

Bariatric Surgery:

Bariatric surgery is the name given to a variety of surgical procedures that reduce the size of the stomach (mostly) or intestine (sometimes). The stomach is approached through mouth or through keyhole surgery so there is minimal or no incision or scarring.

Bariatric surgery has been the most effective treatment for weight loss and for reducing adverse effects of obesity. It can have significant health benefits in addition to weight loss, including reduction in risk factors for heart disease, fatty liver disease and early death. The blood glucose control achieved in diabetics has been a great additional advantage and allows most of them to stop the diabetes medications – almost amounting to a 'cure' for diabetes.

These sweeping benefits are due to the changes in gut hormones that control hunger and feeling of fullness, in addition to the restricted food intake by a smaller stomach. The weight loss achieved is much more lasting compared to lifestyle changes because the hormonal changes shift the equilibrium towards a lower weight, which can be up to 25% lower than the initial weight.

Drug Therapy:

Given the obesity epidemic ravaging the modern world, inventing a drug to cause significant weight loss (anti-obesity drug) has been the holy grail for the pharmaceutical industry for many decades now. Finally, a ray of hope emerged in 2010s with a class of drugs known as Gliflozins. But this ray never became bright sunshine for the weight-loss hopefuls because these drugs achieved a modest 3-4 kg reduction, though the risk of related chronic diseases did go down.

Eventually, researchers pursuing more effective antidiabetic (blood glucose lowering) drugs found significant weight loss as a positive side effect of a particular class of drugs known as Glutides. These act on a particular receptor in the body that suppresses appetite and reduces food intake, by making the stomach empty slower and giving a signal of fullness to the brain. These drugs achieved 15% weight loss on an average over almost a year – which is almost 5 times of what one can achieve by lifestyle changes alone. There however were some negatives, like once weekly injections (now a daily tablet version is also available), and side effects like nausea, digestive discomfort, loss of muscle mass etc. - many more are now being discovered as doctors gain more experience with these drugs. Also, the weight loss lasts only as long as you take the drug.

This initial breakthrough has been followed by newer drugs that act on 2 receptors (20% weight loss) and 3 receptors (25% weight loss). This comes close to what you can expect from Bariatric surgery, though it will reverse when you stop the drug.

It is expected that in future we will be able to control our weight by just popping a daily pill - as we do today for blood pressure and blood sugar. Let's pray for that future to arrive sooner...!

8.

Exercise to lose weight...

Wrong!

This might come as a surprise to you. We have been led to believe that we must exercise to lose weight. Popular media including films, TV serials and reality shows have actively perpetuated this myth by showing actors huffing and puffing and losing weight.

Common sense also leads us to the impression that we can lose weight by burning more calories and exercise is the instrument to do just that. It is also common for people to exercise longer today to burn off extra calories consumed the previous day.

Can you really lose weight by burning more calories during exercise? Well, biology is not as mathematical as that!

We don't realise how incredibly efficient our bodies are. How many calories do you burn during one hour of walk? Same as you get in one banana! If you walk very briskly, maybe 2 bananas. That's all.

Someone might argue that walking is too mild an exercise and therefore more intense exercises like running, cycling, Pilates or fast aerobics will burn more calories and therefore lead to weight loss.

Once again, we don't realise that it is not the calories burned during exercise, but the calories burned over 24 hours that count. Recall the first chapter: body compensates and resists change. When you burn a lot of extra calories during exercise, the body tries to compensate for that by slowing down the metabolism for the rest of the day. This makes the body burn less calories in other functions. It slows you down, makes you sleep more, eat more and digest faster, thus trying to compensate the extra calories lost.

In 2021 researchers compared the effects of different types of exercise on fat loss by analysing 56 studies. They found that the amounts of fat lost due to the exercise itself weren't that significant when done alone without dietary changes: People who exercised more also ended up eating more calories, thus compensating the extra calories burned.

If you have never exercised and you start exercising, initially you may lose a few kilos. But after that your weight becomes constant. You expect your weight to keep going down because you are burning extra calories every day! When that does not happen, many give up in frustration.

For losing weight, one has to reduce the overall 24-hour calorie intake by changing the type and quantity of food. One cannot lose weight by exercise alone.

Then why exercise at all? Exercise one must, for the following benefits, not just for losing weight:

- As already explained, exercise lowers the inflammation, which in turn lowers the risk of various chronic diseases like heart disease, high blood pressure, diabetes, thyroid disorder, sleep disorders, arthritis, cancer etc.
- Exercise triggers autophagy as already discussed. This recycles cellular wastes and rejuvenates the cells, thus slowing down cellular aging.
- Not only on the body, but exercise also has beneficial effect on the brain and psychology. It can prevent and even reverse dementia, depression and anxiety. It also helps stabilise mood and maintain motivation.
- Exercise improves physical strength, stamina, posture and bone health.
- Improved blood and oxygen circulation improves health of all the organs.
- All these effects combine to slow down aging and delay age related problems.

Improved physical strength is one of the most underrated effects of exercise, because people exercise either to lose weight or to build visible muscles. However, many studies have shown that physical strength is a strong predictor of positive health and conversely physical weakness is a predictor of negative health outcomes. So much so, that now there is a debate in the medical community to include 'grip strength' (a measure of one's physical strength) as a vital sign in addition to the traditional body temperature, weight, heart rate, and blood pressure!

Another study found that low physical strength is correlated with faster ageing at the cellular level.

Here are the health risks associated with low physical strength:

- Diabetes
- Heart disease
- Cancer
- Osteoporosis (weak bones)
- Depression
- Dementia / Alzheimer's disease
- Premature death from any cause

This should be the reason to exercise, not weight loss. Is it not reason enough...?

9.

Exercise speeds up metabolism...

Not Always!

This is another common belief when it comes to exercise benefits: once we start exercising, our metabolic rate will remain permanently elevated, thus burning off more calories and making us lose weight.

Nothing could be farther from truth. As already discussed in previous chapter, the body can compensate any extra calories burned during exercise and tries to keep your 24-hour calorie consumption constant.

It is not uncommon for people who have never exercised in their life to suddenly start exercising (mostly on medical advice) and then expecting that now all will be well. People who have been sedentary all their lives suddenly start morning/evening walks and expect miracles. Most of them soon get frustrated and give up. If you start exercising for the wrong reason, you will stop for the wrong reason, and will miss out on all the other benefits that come with it.

Yes, indeed exercise can increase your metabolic rate but only when it leads to an increase in muscle mass, like weights training, resistance training or yoga. And it does not happen immediately; the results start showing themselves after 3 to 6 months. Your brain, your nerves, your hormones, your bones, ligaments, tendons etc. – all have to adapt before your muscles can get bigger. This is one more reason why people give up – they expect immediate visible results and get frustrated when they don't see a change in their bodies. Remember this – the invisible parts of your body have to change before the visible parts can – and that takes time.

Ensure adequate protein intake when you engage in such workouts. Also remember that your frame size has a bearing on how much muscle mass you can gain – as already discussed earlier. Keep your expectations realistic. Bigger muscles, even if not strikingly visible, will burn more calories and absorb more of the blood glucose even at rest. Exercise for health, not just for vanity...!

10.

So cardio is not important...?

It absolutely is!

From the previous chapter, you might have got the impression that the only kind of exercises that increase the muscle mass are the important ones. What of the other kind - the cardiovascular exercises, popularly known as 'cardio'?

Any kind of activity that makes you huff and puff, i.e., makes you breathe heavily and increases your heart rate significantly and keeps it that way for at least 45 minutes, increases your cardio-respiratory fitness (improves functioning of your heart and lungs). Such exercises are known as 'vigorous' or 'high intensity'. Even weights training will increase your heart and breath rate, but only for short periods at a time. Experts opine that to get the optimum health advantage out of cardio the activity must be continued for at least 45 minutes. Of course, a high intensity activity like running or full speed cycling cannot be continued for 45 minutes at a stretch, so you can alternate between high and medium intensity as per your endurance but must continue the activity for at least 45 minutes. This even applies to brisk walking for at least 45 minutes. But doing a 10-minute jog/run as a warm-up before weights training does not count as cardio.

What counts as intense or vigorous activity? The biggest muscles in our body are those of hips and upper legs. Exercises that involve these muscles put sufficient load on the heart and can count as intense or vigorous. Therefore, brisk walking, jogging, running, squats, lunges, push-ups, swimming, speed cycling, skipping etc. are all ok. But if you don't move these muscles at all then moving the rest of the body would not be of much consequence.

All the benefits of exercise discussed earlier apply to cardio as well. Just to summarise once again:

- Cardio-respiratory fitness reduces the risk of almost all chronic diseases, particularly of cardiovascular disease that leads to heart attack or stroke.
- Improves blood sugar and blood pressure control, improves blood circulation and reduces inflammation.
- Has positive psychological effects (mood, motivation).
- Induces autophagy and slows down ageing.

Current guidelines from the World Health Organization and the American Heart Association recommend at least

150 minutes of MVPA (moderate-to-vigorous physical activity) weekly to lower risk for cardiovascular disease and death. This can pretty well be done over a weekend – as per latest research, without loss of affect.

People with large frames and big bodies find it difficult to do cardio because it requires that much more effort to move a heavier body. On the other hand, they gain muscle mass easily when they do weights. On the opposite end of the spectrum, people with smaller frames have low body weight and find it easy to engage in cardio while not gaining much visibly from weights training. Due to these natural reasons, people tend to gravitate towards one kind of exercise or another. This however is not an optimal way to get the full benefit out of the different kinds of exercise. The best strategy is to do both on alternate days. One day for cardio and one for day weights – mixing both on the same day is not advisable because the body needs time to recover. Or you can also do cardio over the weekends, as per the research already mentioned.

The impact of weights training is visible by way of bulging muscles and increased strength. Is the impact of cardio perceptible? Yes indeed - by way of lower 'resting heart rate'. This is the number of times your heart beats per minute while you are at rest. Normally it is between 60-100, but as cardio exercise improves the efficiency of the heart-lung system, it can do the same job with less effort. Therefore, the resting heart rate is lowered. A well-trained athlete or mountain climber can have a resting heart rate as low as 40.

To comprehend the significance of this, consider the following: Mammals live for 1 billion heartbeats. A rabbit's heart beats faster, so its life is short – around 3 years. Elephant's heart beats slower, so it can live for up to 80 years. Lower resting heart rate therefore translates into longer lifespan or slower ageing!

A recent study shows that cardio-respiratory fitness is associated with up to 40% lower risk of 9 types of cancer.

Another reason why cardio is important: Exposure to open sky and green spaces has its own beneficial effect on the body and mind.

Yes of course, you can also do it on a treadmill, but the biomechanics of walking/running on a treadmill is not the same as our natural one and you also miss out on the outdoor exposure. Heading out...?

11.

Eating small, frequent meals boosts metabolism...

Little scientific evidence!

This is another of those myths circulating on social media: eating small frequent meals boosts metabolism and therefore helps you lose weight.

The origin of this idea lies perhaps in the diet regimen of elite athletes, who need a near constant blood sugar level for optimal performance in competitive sports and therefore eat frequent small meals. This neither allows their blood sugar to go low (as in long gap between meals) nor makes it go very high (as with large meals). Some smart fellows connected the dots in reverse and assumed that these athletes have these great bodies because they eat small frequent meals.

As already discussed, your metabolism is a function of your body composition (frame size, muscle mass, body fat etc.), not your meal plan. Thus, eating small frequent meals may not boost your metabolism, but it certainly can backfire if you are one of those who can't stop once they start. You will end up eating more and gaining weight instead of losing it. Ultimately it is all about the total calories you consume in 24 hours, no matter how you slice and dice it.

In case of diabetics, who are already deficient in insulin, the frequent eating can put extra demand on the already insufficient insulin supply and can therefore mess up their blood glucose control. This becomes even more complicated when the patient takes insulin injections.

It can be helpful to some extent for those who are habituated to eating large meals or those who feel hungry shortly after eating. In these cases, the small sizes take care of portion control, and the frequent eating takes care of hunger pangs. Apart from that, there is little scientific evidence that this kind of eating has any significant benefits over the traditional three meal a day pattern. Besides, if you are a working person, you can't really manage to eat this way. Eating on the job, anyone...?

12.

Can build muscles and lose fat at the same time…

False!

I have seen youngsters who work out in the morning, go for a protein shake, skip breakfast, take a small lunch and then a skimpy low-fat dinner - all in an effort to 'get in shape', which is supposed to mean gaining muscle mass and losing fat at the same time.

Can you really do that? It sounds quite intuitive because muscle and fat convey an opposite set of attributes to our mind. So, gain of one should go along with the loss of another. Therefore, exercise and take protein to build muscles and do away with everything else to lose fat. Sounds logical? But it's not biological.

Building muscles is an anabolic (building up) process. Losing fat is a catabolic (breaking down) process. These processes are induced and maintained by two different sets of hormones in the body which are mutually exclusive i.e., when one is present the other is not. Therefore, the body can either be in an anabolic state or a catabolic state - it cannot be in both the states at once!

When you are trying to gain muscle mass, you have to eat sufficient calories to keep the body in an anabolic state so that it can 'build' muscles, which involves synthesising muscle proteins from the food you eat. The raw material for that is of course protein but it takes sufficient blood sugar levels to switch this machine on. This may lead to some weight and fat gain initially but eventually the increased muscle mass will take care of the extra calories.

When you are trying to lose fat, you restrict your calorie intake to keep the body in a catabolic state so that it will break down fat (and also muscle) and convert the same into calories. Yes, you will lose both fat and muscle, and the proportion will depend on the proportion you have in the body. If there is lots of fat and little muscle, then a lot of fat will be burned and a little muscle. If the other way round, then you will burn a lot of muscle. That is the reason bodybuilders have to eat sufficient calories (not only protein) just to maintain the muscle mass, otherwise the body starts digesting the muscles!

Now you know why you can't do both at the same time.

Actors, models, professional bodybuilders etc. go through a stepwise process before they show themselves off to the world. They first build muscles (and fat) by exercising and keeping the body in an anabolic state. Once they have bulked up sufficiently, they continue the exercise and protein consumption but cut down on other calories to burn fat while minimising muscle loss (it's always there, never zero). At the end of this process, they beget the body you see in photographs and films. You see only the end result, not the intermediate steps, and then try to go to that end result - directly.

Ever tried pumping the accelerator and the break of your car at the same time? You will stay where you are. That's what happens when you mix dieting with bodybuilding...!

13.

Exercise = Sweating...

Not always!

We discussed earlier what an intense exercise looks like: any activity that makes you huff and puff, increases your heart rate and makes you breathe faster. Such activity mostly involves working against some kind of resistance like weights or elastic bands and/or vigorously working the large muscles like hip and upper legs.

But there are those who equate intensity with perspiration! The more you sweat the better the exercise. No sweat: useless or boring exercise. Some intuitively believe that they will lose weight when they sweat, otherwise not. The more they sweat, the faster the weight loss.

Using sweat as a surrogate for the efficacy of exercise may sound like common sense, but like so many other commonsensical myths discussed in this book, it is just that.

Vigorous exercise increases blood circulation to our muscles (making the heart work harder) to supply more oxygen and other nutrients for increased energy expenditure. This increases the body temperature, which makes us sweat. Sweating is the body's mechanism to cool itself - evaporation of the water on our skin causes cooling. It's a defence mechanism because high temperatures can damage the cells.

Therefore, typically weights or cardio exercises will cause sweating. Other exercises like yoga may not - but that does not make them useless.

Falsely equating exercise efficacy with sweating makes people do strange things. I have seen some people walking or jogging with their jackets on, even in hot weather!

Overdressing during exercise to induce sweating can backfire because it defeats the body's defence mechanism for cooling itself. The cooling happens only when the sweat is exposed to the air to allow evaporation. Otherwise, your body temperature will rise, making you sweat even more. Too much sweating can dehydrate you and also cause electrolytes (salt) loss - a negative for your health and stamina.

You may see some weight loss after a hyper -sweaty exercise session or two. This is not real weight loss because it is due to the loss of water from the body, which it will soon regain. It is not fat loss.

So don't bother about sweating. It's a byproduct, not the main product of your exercise. And it is not even necessary. Keep those jackets for winter...!

14.

Spot-fat reduction...

Does not happen!

An overweight middle-aged gentleman walks into the gym and asks the trainer to help him get rid of his bloated midriff. Soon he is belly up on the floor doing crunches. Later you can see him swaying and twisting. This goes on for a month, after that the guy is not to be seen in the gym. He is gone because his belly hasn't.

Building muscles is a mechanical process. When you repeatedly load a muscle, it develops microscopic tears or breaks under the strain of the exercise. When we rest and sleep, our body repairs this muscle - as an adaptive response it makes the muscle stronger than before. This is how your muscles get bigger and stronger as you exercise. That is why you feel soreness (typical dull pain on using the muscle) after some time when you exercise a particular muscle, particularly after a sleep. This pain is due to the pressure exerted on the nerve fibres by the nutrients accumulating in the muscle to carry out the repairs. Also note the importance of sleep in this process.

Burning fat on the other hand is a chemical process. Fat is used by the body as an alternative fuel when the main fuel (glucose) is in short supply. This short supply may be caused by increased demand (exercise/exertion) or decreased supply (dietary restriction/fasting). The shortage of glucose makes the body change its hormonal status so that it starts burning stored fat (and muscle) for fuelling itself. This happens for the entire body, not in a particular part alone.

This is the reason why you can build muscles in a particular part of the body, but you cannot burn fat in a particular part of your body. In other words, you can't reduce fat from a particular spot just by exercising that spot. Of course, increased blood circulation to a particular part will help burn more fat from that part, but that will be a very small impact and even this will happen only when the body is in the fat burning state.

Instead of focusing your attention on a few vanity spots, it is better to get in overall shape by focusing on an exercise program that works for the entire body. And for getting rid of fat from a particular spot, there is no shortcut, except surgery.

As of today, surgery is the only way to remove fat from a particular spot. Better go for that instead of torturing yourself by crunching, twisting and turning. But remember - the void created by surgery will soon be filled again if you don't take care of your lifestyle...!

15.

Joints will be damaged by exercise...

Sports, not exercise!

A common refrain against running is that it will wear out the knee joints. It is generally believed that running puts more load on the joints than standing or walking and therefore it will increase the risk of arthritis.

On the other hand, a 2018 study found that marathon runners had lower instances of arthritis compared to the general population. And marathon is the most extreme kind of running!

Yet another study found that competitive runners had higher rates of arthritis than recreational runners. It seems competition is bad for health in more ways than one!

In general, exercise has controlled and measured movements which is good for joints while competitive sports, which have sudden, jerky or over-exerted movements - are bad for joints. This is the reason why sports related joint injuries are so common.

Studies have shown that the repeated loading of joints through exercise makes the cartilage (shock absorbing soft layer at the end of bones) thicker as an adaptive response and therefore more resistant to wear & tear. The extra mechanical strain created by exercise also makes the ligaments (fibrous tissue joining bone to bone around the joints) stronger and thus improves the stability of the joints.

Exercise makes muscles stronger. Strong muscles protect joints from stress & strain by absorbing shocks, while weak muscles transmit the shocks to the joint. Exercise also reduces inflammation in general, which also protects the joints and delays the onset of arthritis.

Yoga is particularly effective for joints because it improves muscle strength as well as joint flexibility.

However, all this is true only when these exercises are performed with correct posture and technique. Bad posture/technique can damage the joints instead of strengthening them. Also, we have to load the joints progressively so that the adaptive response has the time to work. Sudden loading will put more strain than the joints can handle and lead to damage. Even generally beneficial practices like yoga have to be structured in a way that load/stretch the joints progressively and therefore, practising under a qualified trainer is in order. It is very common to see people who have never exercised to suddenly start something and then end up with back or knee problems.

One should be particularly cautious with exercises involving the spine because most of us with sedentary lifestyles already have bad postures. Loading the spine suddenly with strenuous exercises like weighted squats or *surya namaskar* should be avoided. These should be started only after proper conditioning and with expert supervision.

But of course, if you are grossly overweight then you must bring down the weight through diet before engaging in activities that put load on your joints, particularly the knee joint. Otherwise, your weight damages the joints and the activity gets the blame.

Those who play sports and also exercise - their potential for injury is much lower than those who only play sports. The reason is obvious: exercise conditions their joints to better handle the jerks and exertions of competitive sports. Play to win, but first exercise to play...!

16.

Fit Body = Six Pack...

Not Necessarily!

Our abdominal muscles (technically known as rectus abdominis) are among the hardest-working muscles in the body, connecting the rib cage to the front of the pelvis. These are involved in nearly every movement of the body, keep the body stable and balanced, protect the spine against bending backwards and keeps our internal organs in place by providing a firm abdominal wall.

But that is not what makes the sturdy rectus abdominis so popular. What makes it so is the bevy of models and film stars sporting these muscles as a trophy of ultimate fitness, known as 'abs' or 'six pack' - the latter referring to the shrink-wrapped pack of six cans of beer, to which its undulating surface bears visual resemblance.

We all have this muscle, but in almost every case other than those models and actors, it is hidden beneath a layer of fat of varying thickness and shape (quilt, mattress, pillow...). Making it visible therefore requires removal of this layer of fat. Unfortunately, this fat layer follows the 'first in – last out' system. It is the first to come when you gain weight and the last to go when you lose it. Contrary to popular perception, visible six pack is more about low fat than about strong muscles, and therefore has nothing to do with fitness or stamina or even health.

Social media is full of such imagery and of advisory to achieve the same. Some of the youngsters easily get smitten by this abs-bug and are ready go to any length to get their own 'packs'. Many think they can do it just by exercising more. A certain celebrity is rumoured to have gotten there by doing 100 crunches a day. The reality, however, is entirely different.

Getting these so-called six packs (it can be 4,6 or 8 actually) is a two-pronged process. First, work on the abs so that they become bigger and bulge – this is the easier part. Then, lose fat through a strict diet regimen. The pack becomes visible when you have less than 10% fat in the body. This is an extreme condition and requires strict diet and great discipline.

Let us understand what happens when our body fat percentage goes as low as that. Recall the very first chapter of this book – the body tries to compensate and resist. More so when your survival seems to be at stake. And having very low bodyfat triggers all the survivalist alarm bells, because to the body it appears as if you are starving. Therefore, it tries to slow down the metabolism to the bare minimum.

The body may try to shut down all systems that are not necessary for survival such as your reproductive system, leading to infertility. In fact, studies have shown that 12% of infertility cases are due to low body fat. Body fat plays a significant role in reproduction. Sex hormones are fat soluble, and they are stored in the body's fat layers.

The body thus goes to extremes to conserve calories: your heart rate, blood pressure and blood sugar - all go down. This makes you sleepy, lethargic and feel low energy all the time. You feel constant hunger pangs and cravings for sweet/high calorie food – hence the need for great discipline.

The impact on the brain is particularly serious. Our brain consumes 20% of our calories – when the supply of these is low, the result is brain fog, lack of concentration, bad mood and low motivation. None of this is conducive to optimum performance when you are a student or an intellectual worker.

Obviously, nobody can maintain this level of physique permanently. Even models, actors, bodybuilders etc. can achieve this level only for a short period of time –few months at a time. This is when they get themselves photographed shirtless, not otherwise. And you think they have always looked this way. Now you know that it has nothing to do with fitness or health – it is an extreme condition that is not natural to our body.

When Sylvester Stallone was shooting for Rocky, he was in similar condition. Afterall, he had to sport the rocky physique with six packs and more! While shooting on the set, he found it difficult to concentrate, felt dizzy and drowsy. He had to drink 20 cups of black coffee a day to keep himself awake and do handstands to make blood flow into his head!

If you are one of those who live off their bodies, then all this is ok. But if your place in this world depends on your mental faculties, then this game is not for you...!

17.

The more I exercise, the better...

Not a linear relationship!

'Too much of a good thing...' is almost a cliché, and physical exercise is in no way immune to it. Either motivated by its health benefits or smitten by the vanity of a sculpted physique, men and women, particularly the young ones, routinely overdo the gym routine.

I have seen some gym-rats regularly working out up to 3 hours at a time. I have seen folks running for one hour and then gymming for another one hour. One is certainly impressed by their hard work and dedication, but unfortunately it is in the wrong direction.

After a point, exercise increases inflammation instead of decreasing it. This happens when the body does not get sufficient rest or time to recover from the previous bout of workout. What happens to be too much for you depends on your ability to recover, which in turn is dictated by your physical history and your genes. Professional athletes can recover much faster and therefore can take on much more exercise – but then that is precisely the reason why they are the professional athletes and not you and me!

The increased inflammation due to a cumulative lack of recovery can actually increase the risk of heart disease, stroke and other chronic diseases.

If you are not a pro-athlete, limit your period of any particular intense activity (running, weights training etc.) to one hour per day (at a time) or 3 hours per week (total).

In weights training, beginners should limit to one muscle group a day to allow proper recovery. Also, avoid doing push and pull exercises on the same day so that your supporting muscles also get proper rest. Push exercises are those in which you push the weights away from the body, such as shoulder, chest, triceps. Pull exercises are those in which you pull the weights towards your body, such as back, biceps, deadlifts.

Remember – your objective is to exercise for health, so do not start playing 'mirror-mirror on wall' and following all kinds of tips and tricks circulating on social media, which are mostly for the pros and by the pros.

It's important to have a balanced and well-rounded exercise routine that suits your fitness level and health conditions. If you have any kind of health issues or medical conditions, it's advisable to consult a medical professional before starting any new exercise regimen.

Finally, do net get overly impressed by the great bodies you see in your gym. There may not be any cause-and-effect relationship between what they look like and what they do in the gym. Great bodies are made, as much by the genes and as much in the kitchen as in the gym...!

18.

Women's exercise = Men's exercise...

No; men & women are equal - not identical!

A recent Newsweek report says "Historically, women have been underrepresented in clinical trials and health-based research. Fitness guidelines, it turns out, are no different."

While giving full credit to the equal status of women in the society, we cannot ignore the fact that women and men are built differently, particularly when it comes to physical activity.

Male and female bodies differ in their function, structure and hormones. However, in gym you can witness both doing mostly the same kind of exercises when it comes to weights training. The gym trainers are predominantly male as of today and most of them make both men and women do the same exercises. Can't blame them – that's how they have been trained.

Here is a summary of how different the female and male bodies are and why this should change the way they exercise:

- Females have smaller muscles, smaller upper bodies, finer bones and smaller lungs. Thus, their weight bearing capacity is lower. Also, they have 1/10th of the hormones necessary for muscle gains. Therefore, their bodies do not respond to weights training as fast as the male body does.Overloading can deny them the benefits of exercise and even result in injury.
- Female muscles develop less power but take longer to get tired, and also need more time to recover once tired. Therefore, their regimen should involve more repetitions with smaller weights, longer rests and longer gaps between exercising the same muscle groups.
- Males typically focus more on their arms and upper bodies. Females should focus more on their core and lower body to get the same benefit from their workouts.
- Cardiovascular disease is more common in men – therefore they benefit more by doing cardio. Arthritis is more common in women – so they benefit more by doing yoga. Mother Nature also supports your cause: larger lungs of men make cardio easier for them, while more flexible bodies of women make yoga easier for them.

Young men typically join gyms to increase their muscle mass. Which is ok for them as they have the necessary hormones, and the bigger muscles will take care of their metabolic rate in future. So, they are sorted.

But most young women hit the gym assuming they will burn more calories and get slimmer. This doesn't work without dietary changes - as already discussed earlier. Moreover, most gym trainers typically make them do the same things as men, for which most ladies are not built. No wonder, many drop out due to frustration or injury or both.

Once again, I repeat, particularly for women this time: exercise for the health benefits, not for losing weight. Weights training reduces inflammation, prevents chronic diseases, makes bones and joints stronger, increases protein synthesis which also benefits your skin and hair. Cardio slows down aging. Yoga prevents arthritis, corrects posture and does a lot more...!

19.

Yoga is slow and boring...

So is education!

When you witness people doing yoga, especially the beginners, it appears rather slow and boring. Many, for whom it can be potentially beneficial, stay away from it for this reason. But consider this: even education was boring when we got started. Today we look back and feel fortunate that we ever got one. As Aristotle said, 'The roots of education are bitter, but the fruit is sweet.'

Yoga is not only about physical activity (*asanas*), but also involves breathing exercises (*pranayama*), cleansing techniques (*kriyas*) and meditation (*dhyana*). The most visible and popular aspect however remains the physical aspect of it, which is the poses or *asanas*.

It is widely credited with numerous health benefits, such as reduced inflammation and stress, improved flexibility, better posture, and enhanced mental focus. While most people practice yoga for its physical benefits, its original purpose was to help humankind achieve greater self-awareness and inner peace. *(Those interested in the subject of self-awareness may read my first book: 'Why Buddha Left Home : A scientific guide to self-awareness', available on Amazon, Flipkart etc.)*

The West has developed its own version of yoga by incorporating more speed and physicality into it, turning it almost into a competitive sport. Many tend to prefer this over the traditional practice. However, one should get started on the traditional version to condition the body properly before going for the more physically demanding versions. Without proper guidance, posture correction supervision and progressive loading, even something as benign as yoga can lead to injuries.

In today's fast-paced world, most people expect quick and dramatic results from their workouts, esp. weight loss – about which we have already discussed. Yoga's benefits on the other hand are mostly internal, invisible and accrue over a period of time. Those who prefer high-intensity activities view yoga as too slow-paced or not challenging enough. Some who consider only fast paced exercise as effective tend to discount the efficacy of yoga.

Thus, the benefits of yoga are quite underrated, but here is a summary: Yoga poses combine contraction of one set of muscles and stretching of the opposing muscles. The muscles being contracted gets stronger, due to increased tension. The muscles being stretched produce an anti-inflammatory effect. The stress and strain stimulate the bones, ligaments and joints to get stronger and more resilient. The effort involved in maintaining the poses gently loads and benefits the cardiovascular system as well. Thus, the overall benefits are reduced inflammation, better strength, joint mobility and improved circulation. All this translates into reduced risk of arthritis and other chronic diseases.

Also, if you have a health condition then yoga has specific instructions in terms of *asanas* and variations that you should and should not do. There is a practice called 'therapeutic yoga' to help you manage your specific health problem.

The perception that yoga is always slow is also not true. Once you cross the beginner level and if you are fit enough, there are various levels of challenging and fast paced series of interrelated poses known as *vinyasa* flows. Some of these can leave even the fittest in sweat. Even US Marines, who are among the toughest soldiers on earth, are now being trained on yoga.

There is one more benefit that is unique to yoga: posture correction. Yoga practice over a period of time corrects your posture even without your conscious awareness of it.

We don't realise how important posture is for our health and personality. Most of us have bad postures, having started our lives hunched on our textbooks, followed by office desks and screens. Towards the middle age, the battle of the bulge begins. The growing belly shifts our centre of gravity forward and our spine has to work extra hard to keep the balance, leading to low back pain and other back problems. The body's systems being interconnected, bad posture in turn affects the joints, the digestive system and the respiratory system among others. It affects how you stand and how you walk, and thus your personality.

In the West there is a professional called Chiropractor who specialises in posture correction. We don't have that in India, but thank God we have yoga...!

20.

Take exercise supplements...

Only after fact-checking!

Weights training leads to muscle repair and growth, for which protein is the key raw material. While non-vegetarians can possibly consume sufficient protein through their diet itself, vegetarian diet is typically low in protein, and they may need to take a protein supplement to cover the deficit.

Gym trainers routinely advise people to take a whey protein supplement as a protein shake. It is ok to take 30gm (1 scoop typically) per day. Taking in excess can overload your liver and kidneys. It is best to consult a doctor before starting any supplement to ensure you are a good candidate for the same, especially if you are over 35. The best time is to take it is within one hour of finishing your workout, because at this time the body is more primed for protein absorption.

However, the market is full of all kinds of varieties of whey protein. Do your own fact-checking before going after the brand/product you are being advised or sold and make sure the manufacturer is trustworthy. Here is a summary of various kinds of whey protein products available:

- Whey Protein Concentrate (WPC): This contains a moderate level of protein (typically around 70-80%) along with some fat and carbohydrates. It also retains some of the beneficial nutrients found in whole whey, so this is a more wholesome product.
- Whey Protein Isolate (WPI): WPI is a more refined form, with a higher protein content (around 90%) and lower levels of fat and carbohydrates. It a popular choice for those looking to minimize calorie intake.
- Whey Protein Hydrolysate (WPH): This is hydrolysed, which breaks down the protein into smaller peptides. This makes the protein easier to digest and can potentially reduce the risk of allergic reactions if someone is allergic to cow's milk. But it is absorbed fast so should not be taken in large doses at a time.
- Plant Proteins: These may include pea protein, rice protein, hemp protein etc. While not as effective as whey protein, they offer a plant-based alternative for those who want to avoid animal products or are allergic to milk/lactose.
- Blends: Some products offer a blend of different types of whey protein. It may include whey protein concentrate, isolate, and hydrolysate in varying

proportions. The idea is to provide a combination of fast-acting and long-acting proteins.

- Specialised Formulas: In addition to these, you may find specialised formulas designed for specific purposes. These could include post-workout recovery blends, meal replacement shakes, weight loss blends etc. These may include additional ingredients like vitamins, minerals or herbal extracts. Here you have to be particularly careful about the ingredients as some may be potentially harmful.

If not sure, just go for the simple whey protein concentrate from a good manufacturer. To avoid artificial sweeteners and flavours, you can go for the unsweetened and unflavoured versions. These are more natural but are bland in taste, which you can improve by adding some fruit and milk.

Another supplement that is considered safe is HMB (hydroxy methyl butyrate). Research suggests it may help reduce muscle breakdown and promote muscle repair. A recent study found that HMB can prevent brain damage in Alzheimer's disease. It is generally safe and well tolerated in the dose range of 1 to 3 gm per day. In rare cases, people may experience stomach pain, constipation, or itching.

In addition to these, you may be advised potentially harmful supplements by those who wish to impress you by showing quick results. Here is a summary of harmful supplements/drugs one should avoid:

- Creatine: It helps maintain a continuous energy supply to muscles during intense exercise. It may help increase muscle growth and speed up recovery. While generally considered safe and effective, excessive use or high doses can lead to dehydration and kidney damage.
- Anabolic Steroids: These are synthetic variations of testosterone, the male hormone. They increase muscle mass, but have serious health risks, including liver damage, cardiovascular issues, hormonal imbalances, and psychological effects.
- Prohormones: These are precursors to hormones, including testosterone. They are marketed as natural alternatives to steroids, but they can still pose similar risks to liver and heart health.
- Androstenedione (Andro): This was once a popular supplement believed to boost testosterone levels. However, it was found to have little to no benefit and could potentially increase the risk of heart disease and hormone imbalances.
- Growth Hormone Releasing Peptides (GHRPs): These can increase muscle mass, but can have adverse effects on insulin sensitivity, potentially leading to diabetes.
- DMAA (Dimethylamylamine): This stimulant was found in some pre-workout supplements and was

associated with increased heart rate, high blood pressure, and even strokes. It has been banned in some countries.

- Clenbuterol: It promotes fat loss. However, it can lead to serious cardiovascular and metabolic side effects.
- Ephedra: This herbal supplement was commonly used for weight loss and energy enhancement. However, it has been banned in many countries due to its association with severe cardiovascular events and even death.
- Liver Support Supplements: Ironically, some supplements marketed as liver support can themselves be harmful. They may contain ingredients that are toxic to the liver.
- Unregulated Supplements: Some products may contain undisclosed harmful ingredients, especially those from unreliable sources. A recent study in US found that 40% of sports supplements selling online including herbal ones either did not contain the listed ingredient, contained wrong amount of one or more ingredients and some even had illegal/banned additives. Therefore, always go for reputable manufacturers, if at all.

Another important thing to note is that a particular supplement alone may be ok in a particular dose, but when combined with another supplement, it may turn toxic. Therefore, before taking any new supplement, it's important to consult a healthcare professional. If you are on medications or have preexisting health conditions, then this is a must.

It is equally important to do your own research and see whether the tips and advice you receive hold scientific merit. It is tragic to learn every now and then of someone ending up with kidney or liver damage after taking an exercise or sports supplement. Over-ambitious youngsters keen to build impressive bodies or to win medals routinely fall for such traps...!

21.

Take multivitamin everyday...

Can be toxic!

It is commonly understood that the multivitamins are supposed to be taken every day. This is how doctors prescribe them and some even have this mentioned on their label.

What is not commonly understood is that the once daily dose is a 'therapeutic dose'. In simple terms this means it is for those who are sick, are suffering nutritional deficiencies due to malnutrition or malabsorption, or are very old.

If you are otherwise healthy and eating normally, then you don't need the therapeutic dose. All you need is a maintenance dose, which can be once or twice a week. In some cases, like high dose vitamin D, it can even be once a month.

Why take the maintenance dose at all? Because we might be somewhat lacking in one vitamin or mineral or other, due to our dietary habits or lifestyle. As mentioned earlier, the best way is to eat as much variety as possible. But that is not always possible and therefore taking a multivitamin can protect you from potential deficiencies. For example, vegetarians are usually deficient in vitamins that come only from animal source, such a vitamin B_{12}. Due to limited sunlight exposure, most of us are deficient in vitamin D – which is now implicated in increased inflammation leading to various chronic diseases. It is advisable to get these checked and corrected under medical supervision.

Research has shown mixed results on multivitamin supplementation. Some show no benefit, some show limited benefit. This is because the benefits depend on your nutritional status. If you are already getting enough from your food, then addition of a supplement has no benefit. If your food is deficient in a particular nutrient, then adding that nutrient as a supplement will benefit you. A recent study found that giving a daily multivitamin to the elderly (60+) improved their memory (brain function). Another recent study from AIIMS Bhatinda found that taking a calcium + vitamin D supplement daily did not reduce the risk of fractures. It is common to see such inconsistent results in research on supplements because their calculations cannot include what the study subjects were already getting from their food.

The important thing to note is that we are already getting these vitamins and minerals from the food we eat. The supplement is not the only source. Therefore, if we are eating normally and are otherwise healthy, then taking the once daily dose may cause excess of certain vitamins/minerals and cause toxicity. In general, whenever you take any supplement, give it a break from time to time so as to allow clearance of any possible accumulation and thus prevent potential toxicity.

In India, these supplements are available under various regulatory licenses. There are high dose vitamins and minerals available under drug license, which are for therapeutic use and are supposed to be prescribed by doctors, but prescription is not necessary for sale. This is the category where we have to be more careful about the dose (maintenance dose v/s. therapeutic dose).

Then there are those available under food license as 'nutraceuticals' or nutritional supplements. These are relatively low dose, but not without their own share of potential toxic effects if taken in excess. These can be synthetic chemicals as well as herbal or animal products. As these are under food license, they cannot claim to cure any disease on their label, but most manufacturers still do mention the benefits their product is supposed to provide.

Herbal supplements are also available in India under one of the licenses under the Ministry of AYUSH (Ayurveda, Yoga, Unani, Siddha and Homeopathy). These are allowed to mention therapeutic claims on the pack according to the classical systems of medicine on which the formula is based. These may contain one or more standardised extracts (chemical components extracted from plants) or botanicals (parts of plants).

India being the land of Ayurveda, herbal products and supplements are available aplenty. In popular perception these are safe simply because these are herbal, which is considered the same as being natural. The reality is not as simple as that. There are various question marks when it comes to the quality of commercially available herbal products, especially those which are made from botanicals (plants or parts thereof); those containing standardised extracts are less of a problem:

- Does the botanical really have the health advantage being claimed?
- Does the product actually contain the plant that is being claimed?
- Has the plant been grown and harvested in the ideal conditions that provide the claimed benefit?
- Has the plant not been adulterated with similar looking but useless plants?
- Does the product actually have the labelled quantity of the botanical?
- Has the product been contaminated during processing?
- Have heavy metals leached and entered into the product during solvent extraction or other such processes?

- Is there a way to standardise the biological activity of the product from batch to batch?
- What happens to this activity over a period of time on storage? At what temperature?

With so many questions marks, it is easy to imagine that 'if something can go wrong, it will'. In my experience, it takes much more to develop a standardised herbal product as compared to a synthetic one. Developing and manufacturing such products need special expertise and technologies - one's knowledge of Ayurveda, naturopathy, yoga etc. does not automatically translate into such expertise.

Of course, there are many reputable Indian manufacturers taking care of all these question marks and making highly standardised products and also doing extensive clinical studies to prove their efficacy and safety. Many of these products provide significant benefits and fill therapeutic gaps where allopathy does not have a solution.

It is therefore advisable to seek relevant expert guidance or medical advice before taking any herbal supplement on your own.

Finally, however natural or beneficial a substance or ingredient may be – after a point it can become toxic. Therefore, practice moderation. There is a saying that 'dose is the poison, not the substance'. At high doses, anything can become a poison, even the most beneficial and life-giving substance. Even water becomes toxic if you drink too much – 'water toxicity' is a known medical condition...!

22.

Sugar substitutes are good...

May have side effects!

The World Health Organization (WHO) has recently released a new guideline on non-sugar sweeteners (sugar substitutes or artificial sweeteners). It recommends against the use of these as substitute for sugar, except in case of diabetics.

The recommendation is based on a review of the available evidence which suggests that the use of these substances does not confer any long-term benefit in reducing body fat in adults or children. The review also suggests that there may be potential undesirable effects from their long-term use, such as an increased risk of diabetes, cardiovascular diseases, cancers etc.

Common products in this category include acesulfame K, aspartame, advantame, cyclamates, neotame, saccharin, sucralose, stevia and stevia derivatives.

The recommendation does not apply to personal care and hygiene products, such as toothpaste, skin cream, and medications.

In simpler terms, there is no point in using such products for weight management or calorie restriction, because the risks are greater than the benefits.

The problem is that these substances are not nutrients – these are chemicals that somehow fool our taste buds into giving a signal of sweet taste to the brain. These chemicals are not natural to the body, so some side effects were expected, which have finally been discovered.

A better strategy is to reduce sugar intake gradually, so that you will get used to the less sweet taste. If you add one teaspoon of sugar to your tea/coffee, reduce to 3/4th and after a month or two, to half. You will get used to it.

Another way out is to reduce the consumption of sugary drinks like colas and packaged fruit juices or other fruit flavoured beverages because these come loaded with sugar. And we consume a glass-full of it at a time (you can sip it slowly to reduce the impact). Many of these contain fructose instead of sugar, which gets converted to sugar in the liver. A recent study shows that daily consumption of such beverages can increase the risk of liver diseases, including liver cancer.

It is an irony that people go to great lengths to avoid sugar, but at the same time consume with abandon many snacks that are almost immediately converted to sugar in the body, such as bread, biscuits, doughnuts, bagels, croissants, cornflakes, French fries, potato chips, boiled potato preparations and other easily digestible starchy stuff. Actually, we should name these foodstuff as 'sugar substitutes'...!

23.

Do 'xyz' every day, all problems go away...

Be careful!

Originating in conventional wisdom and amplified by social media, there are widely held beliefs about many activities and remedies that promise good health if done every day. Closer scrutiny however reveals that attaining good health is not as simple as that!

Let us take these on one by one...

The most common one is that taking honey and lemon in warm water every morning will boost your metabolism, burn fat and make you lose weight (irrespective of whatever else you might be doing to your body). There is no scientific basis for that claim.

At the most, if you are skipping breakfast and only consuming this, then the sugar in honey may quell your hunger pangs and the vitamins in honey and lemon may benefit you. But this alone cannot burn your fat. In fact, there is no such magical formula that you can take every day and lose weight, except of course the new weight loss drugs.

Same applies to warm water. It cannot boost your metabolism just because it is warm. Everything comes to body temperature once it reaches the stomach. At the most, it may be good for your throat and may help your bowel movement.

Then there are social media posts telling the virtues of drinking 1 litre of water every morning, promising all your health troubles will go away. Logic? Because 70% of our body is water. Well, 20% of our body is carbon, so eating a piece of coal every morning will help? One litre is a large amount of water for our body and even with normal kidney function, it takes almost an hour to remove the same. For someone with diabetes or high BP, it can disturb the blood sugar or blood pressure. For someone with low kidney function or weak heart, it can be potentially disastrous. Again, there is no scientific basis for such claims. Drinking 2-3 glasses is good for hydration and bowel movement, but no more than that.

There are many such 'health tips' floating around on social media which claim to be sourced from Ayurveda or other such classical sources. It is important to verify the veracity of such claims on two levels – 1. Does it really come from the claimed source? -2. This is really how the original statement is worded or is it just an interpretation? A lot can be open to interpretation when one quotes something written in Sanskrit in the ancient times. When it comes to health, the best policy is to follow information that is based on evidence based research.

Another swift footed idea of our times is that if you walk 10,000 steps every day, all your health issues are taken care of. The number actually came from a marketing campaign for a pedometer device during the 1964 Tokyo Olympics. Since then, it has helped sell numerous such devices and watches that measure your steps. Going by the sales, it may well be one of the most effective marketing campaigns of all times! Is there a scientific basis for this magic number? None! Ideally the more you walk the better, especially if you are not doing any other exercise, but those incremental benefits don't stop at 10,000 steps. According to a recent study, you must walk at least 4000 steps a day for significant reduction in risk of death by any cause (disease). This risk decreases by 15% for every increment of 1000 steps per day. There are no other magic numbers involved.

Then there are many teas/fruits/juices/recipes/formulas being claimed to have the ability to burn belly fat. This we have already discussed – there is no such silver bullet that can single handedly end this belly-battle.

There are many more such tips or hacks or magic formulas going around on social media. I can't cover all of those here, but the idea is to develop a healthy scepticism and fact-check the claims being made in such communications. Do not trust appearances, especially in these times of shallow knowledge and deep fakes. Someone wearing a white coat and glasses may not be a real doctor...!

24.

Eating raw food is healthy…

Up to a point!

Another trend that has caught on in recent times is to favour raw foods diets. Their supposed logic is that modern food is a problem so let's do what our stone age ancestors did – eat raw food.

Well, certain foods are meant to be eaten raw, such as fruits (technically, tomato and cucumber are also fruits) and some tubers like carrots, radishes, turnips, beetroot etc. and of course nuts or dry fruits. These are good for health as we all know but these can be eaten in only limited quantities, otherwise we will have digestive issues.

The original idea was to eat fresh and unprocessed food, instead of processed or frozen food. This idea somehow got stretched into a raw food fad.

First of all, this perception that our ancestor ate raw food is wrong. The prehistoric (ape-like) proto-human ate raw food which had to be cut and chewed with a lot of force, so they had very strong jaw muscles and also very strong digestive system to digest the raw food. Probably by accident, over time they discovered that food exposed to fire tastes very good. This must have led them to start the cooking of food on fire.

The cooked food was easy to chew and easy to digest. Because it was easy to chew, the strong jaw muscles were no longer needed, they weakened over time and no longer required large attachment area on the skull. This allowed the skull to become larger, in turn allowing our brain to become larger. At the same time, as the cooked food was digested easily and faster, so the digestive system became smaller, consumed less calories for itself and made available large number of calories for the bigger brain. These two developments came together to allow us to become the intelligent human (homo sapiens) that we are today. Therefore, it is cooked food that has made us human, and not the other way around.

Therefore, including modest portions of raw fruits, vegetables etc. is good for its nutrient content and because it promotes beneficial gut bacteria that reduce inflammation. It also makes you feel full faster and thus reduces overall calorie consumption. But going entirely raw would be stretching it too far because our digestive systems are not designed to handle so much uncooked material.

We are not built for raw food, instead we have evolved because of cooked food...!

25.

Fruit + vegetable juices are healthy…

Can be dangerous!

Social media and internet sites are full of mixed juice recipes that include fruits and vegetables mixed together to supposedly make them more healthy and lower in calories. Being colourful, these also look quite attractive in Instagram pictures. Many packaged goods companies have started selling such mixed juices to encash the trend.

There are two issues here.

First, if you can chew, juices are not for you. Our bodies evolved while eating fruits and vegetables, not while drinking their juices. The juices overload our system with large amount of nutrients, which is not natural. And if these are filtered or centrifuged, then all those fibres that promote beneficial gut bacteria are being thrown away. It is ok to occasionally take fresh cold pressed juice of those fruits that involve too much labour to eat or are too sour for your teeth, such as citrus fruits and pomegranate.

Secondly, many vegetables are high in oxalate such as spinach, beetroot, carrots and most fruits are high in citric acid, especially the citrus fruits as the name suggests. When you mix these two, the citric acid increases the absorption of oxalate in the body. High levels of oxalate can increase the risk of kidney stones. This is particularly applicable to juices because a large quantity is consumed in a short time, as compared to eating the same.

Therefore, try to eat as far as possible instead of making juices out of fruits and vegetable. And even if you do, do not mix the two.

People have been consuming many other juices out of conventional wisdom. Like the juice of the bottle gourd (*lauki*) is believed to help in weight loss. Yes, it has very little calories and lots of fibre, but it will help only when you replace your normal food with bottle gourd, not when you take the juice in addition to your normal diet! It does not contain any magical ingredient that makes you lose weight. Also, there have been reports of serious infections from raw bottle gourd juice, so take care.

Another favourite gourd of ours is the bitter gourd (*karela*). Diabetics consume its juice because it is supposed to lower blood sugar. Well, there is indeed some truth in it – there is a compound in it that actually has antidiabetic or blood sugar lowering property. But in a six-month toxicity study this compound was found to be toxic to kidneys. Diabetes itself is bad for the kidneys, in addition if you are taking *karela* juice daily, then it's a double whammy for the poor kidney.

This is another example of our erroneous assumption that something is harmless because it is natural. When taken as a juice, you get a large dose at once and this amplifies whatever effects it might have - good, bad or ugly..!

26.

Detox...

Does not work!

Social media and internet are full of detox recipes of all kinds (juices, diets etc.). These are supposed to cleanse or detoxify your body. Do they work? How?

Let us first understand the comings and goings of these so-called toxins in our body.

When we eat, the digested food is absorbed into the blood and first passes through the liver before it could go anywhere else in the body. The liver is a 'chemically intelligent' organ. It knows whether a particular substance is good for the body or not. Those which are bad are broken down until they become water soluble so that these can be removed by the kidney through urine. If any of these broken-down products are fat soluble then these are sent back to the intestine to get removed through the faeces. Some fat-soluble nutrients that can be toxic at high levels in the blood, are stored in the liver and released as and when required.

So, if your liver and kidney are doing their usual jobs, then there is no way any toxin can get stored anywhere in this process, which you would kick out later through a special detox diet. And if your liver and kidney are not doing their job, then anyway you need a doctor urgently – not a detox.

On the contrary, many of those detox formulas that induce diarrhoea or excess urination, may lead to dehydration and electrolyte imbalance, which increase the workload on your liver and kidneys, thus increasing toxicity instead of decreasing it.

Cellular wastes can accumulate inside the cells, but those cannot come out of the cell just because you are in the mood for detox. The cell membrane maintains strict border control on all the atoms and molecules entering or exiting the cell. That is one of the secrets of its survival in this big bad world!

As already discussed earlier under 'autophagy', these wastes get recycled within the cell when the cell is under stress due to nutrient scarcity. And this scarcity can be created either by reduced supply (fasting) or increased demand (exercise). Not by eating or drinking something special...!

27.

Fried food is bad...

If from animal source!

Most people avoid fried food because of its fat content – because they think that fat will get stored in the body. This issue we already clarified very early in this book: it is the total calories that matter, not the type of calories.

Indeed, oils and fats have almost ten times the calories per gram compared to other foods and therefore one should be mindful of the same it trying to lose weight. But fried food is not the only source of fat in Indian cooking; oils and fats are an integral part of the seasoning process (*tadka* or *chhonk*) of dishes that we eat 2-3 times a day. Minimising this part can help you reduce more calories than the occasional fried delicacies you enjoy. Also remember that fats are absorbed slowly and do not raise your blood sugar rapidly. Frying is only a method of cooking – what you are cooking is more important.

The bigger issue with frying is that the food is exposed to very high temperatures, which generates toxic products. This is particularly serious with animal products, like meat, eggs, cheese etc. The same applies to fats from animal source used as a frying medium such as butter and *ghee* (clarified milk fat). Frying in hydrogenated vegetable oils is the worst as it also produces 'trans fats' which are bad for the heart.

Frying vegetable products like grains, seeds, nuts etc. is less of a problem. This is ok in moderation / occasionally. For the same reason oils from vegetable sources are a safer frying medium.

However, there is a debate about which oils are better – refined oils or virgin (unrefined) oils? There are people on both sides of this oil divide, preferring one over the other. Companies selling refined oils promote their low cholesterol and low-calorie virtues. Social media on the other hand is abuzz with the benefits of virgin oils. Who is telling the truth? Both, this time for a change!

Refined oils and virgin oils have the same source (seeds that contain oil) but differ in their processing methods and therefore their properties. Each type has its own set of advantages and disadvantages. Let's compare their pros and cons:

Refined Oils:

Pros:

- Higher Smoke Point: Smoke point is the temperature at which an oil starts burning. Refined oils generally have a higher smoke point, which makes them more suitable for high heat cooking like frying.
- Longer Shelf Life: The refining process removes impurities and free fatty acids, resulting in a longer shelf life and better stability.
- Less Thickness: The refining process removes the waxy or gummy part of the natural oil, making it light and more free flowing.

Cons:

- Nutrient Loss: The refining process involves heat, chemicals and filtration, which can reduce some of the natural nutrients, including antioxidants, vitamins and other fat-soluble nutrients.
- Chemical Residues: Some refined oils may retain traces of the chemicals used during processing, therefore source it from good manufacturers.

Virgin Oils:

Pros:

- Rich Flavour: Virgin oils retain the natural flavours and aromas of the source material, which can enhance the taste.
- Higher Nutritional Value: Since virgin oils undergo minimal processing, they tend to retain more of their

natural nutrients, such as vitamin E, antioxidants, and other beneficial compounds.

Cons:

- Lower Smoke Point: Virgin oils generally have lower smoke points, making them less suitable for high-temperature cooking like frying. They may also form more toxic products when used for frying due to burning of various nutrients.
- Shorter Shelf Life: Due to the presence of natural impurities and free fatty acids, virgin oils generally have a shorter shelf life compared to refined oils.

It should be clear from the above that refined oils are more suitable for frying while virgin oils are more suitable for low heat cooking, salad dressings and pickles. Use both to get the best of both the worlds...!

28.

Spices are bad...

Only in excess !

Some people while dieting avoid spices entirely in the belief that it will help them lose weight faster. Maybe it works by making them eat less of the bland fare. There are others who equate spices with an indulgence and try to minimise it. In India there is a tradition of *satvik* (pious) food that is made without spices with the belief that spices promote impious or impure tendencies of the mind.

Individual beliefs notwithstanding, the fact remains that these are supposed to be used in minute quantities. Spices are pungent and therefore can irritate the valve between the food pipe and stomach, making it relax and allowing the acidic stomach contents to get into the food pipe, giving rise to the burning sensation that we normally call 'acidity'. This term is not only a misnomer as it implies an excess of acid in the stomach, but also makes people try to relieve it by taking antacids. Some cold milk or a banana to soothe the valve would be a more natural remedy, especially because the pungent stuff in the spices is mostly fat soluble. Not lying down soon after eating would be another good idea.

Spices are not just an indulgence of taste. We evolved to like their taste for a reason, just as we evolved to like the taste of high calorie food. Spices must have offered an evolutionary advantage to those who used them, particularly in the hot tropical regions, where they grow naturally and are used extensively. Indeed, modern science also shows that spices have antibacterial, anti-parasite, antioxidant and anti-inflammatory properties, thus preventing acute as well as chronic diseases. Including wide range of spices in the food also provides a variety of micronutrients to the body, which are required in very minute quantities but are important for overall health.

Just like all those things that are good in moderation, spices can cause heartburn in excess, but a little is enough to spice up your life...!

29.

Gluten is bad...

Only for a chosen few !

Gluten is the protein part of wheat – it is the best part if you ask me, because the rest is all carbohydrate, which get absorbed very fast and makes you fat!

However, in the popular perception fuelled by social media and advertising, it has been turned into a villain. It has been made into a 'bad' ingredient that one should avoid.

In reality, it is bad only for those who are allergic to gluten, which is highly unlikely if your ancestors are from North India, Europe or Middle East because wheat has been eaten in these regions for millennia. Anyone with the genes for this kind of allergy would have been removed from the gene pool long ago.

This allergy is mostly found in those whose ancestors never ate wheat, as in Southeast Asia and some native populations of the Americas and the Pacific.

A few could still have the allergy due to some genetic mutation. But if you were allergic to gluten, the symptoms would have been severe enough to force a doctor visit, leading to a diagnosis of the same in your early childhood. The symptoms include abdominal pain, nausea, diarrhoea, which can lead to fatigue and weight loss if consumption is continued.

If you are free from these symptoms, then there is no need to avoid gluten. Gluten free food is therefore not a healthier alternative or of higher quality in any way.

Then there are those who confuse gluten with glutamate. Monosodium glutamate (MSG), also known as Ajinomoto, is added to food products to enhance their flavour, mostly in Chinese food. It is also found naturally in many types of food. High level of glutamate has been associated with headaches, increased blood pressure, inflammation and even psychiatric disorders. It has nothing to do with gluten.

Labelling food as 'gluten free' started in the USA where there is a population of mixed ethnicity, and many did have the allergy. Gradually somehow it became a mark of healthier or superior quality food.

In the Jodhpur area of Rajasthan, the western province of India, they make a dish out of pure gluten. All the carbohydrate is washed off the wheat flour, and the gummy gluten that is left behind is cut into cubes and made into a delicacy. It is consumed with relish on every grand occasion – yet those guys are hale and hearty…!

30.

Vegan is great...

If red meat is the only other option!

Consumption of red meat and processed meat is bad for health as well as the environment. These meats are associated with an increased risk of cancers and other chronic diseases. Raising animals for this meat is a huge source of greenhouse gases, contributing to global warming. In an extreme reaction to this, many (particularly in the West) have turned Vegan, eschewing any food stuff coming from animal source, including milk or eggs.

This is like swinging the pendulum from one extreme to the other. Our bodies have evolved with nutrients coming from both plant and animal sources. This sudden break is not natural.

Many so-called celebrities and influencers claim on social media that they feel great after giving up dairy. Giving up milk and dairy products may help those who have lactose intolerance, but that is unlikely for those with Indian and

European ancestry, where milk has been consumed as a staple for millennia. Another reason why someone may feel 'great' is that dairy products make you feel full and are digested slowly – but as already discussed, that is a good thing!

There are many essential nutrients that predominantly come from animal sources. Research shows that vegans have lower bone density and lower muscle mass (unless they are supplementing with protein). They are also low on Taurine – a nutrient recently found to be associated with longer lifespan or slower ageing.

There are many nutrients that are difficult to obtain from plant sources alone, such as vitamin B_{12}, vitamin D, calcium, omega-3 fatty acids, zinc etc. Therefore, vegans may have to take supplements, which ironically could be coming from animal sources!

Vegans typically use milk substitutes like almond milk; the cultivation and processing of almonds into milk itself has a large water and carbon footprint. So, if the idea is to save the planet, then there isn't much of that happening either.

Our traditional food is a complete ecosystem, with various nutrients coming from various sources and forming a complete package. All you need to do is a little adjustment as per your modern lifestyle. But when you go off these traditions entirely, you create gaps in your nutritional status which you then try to fill up from here and there, further complicating your life…!

31.

Alkaline food / water is better...

Not enough evidence !

This is another fad one comes across these days. Alkaline water or food is being promoted as something that can promote good health or prevent/manage chronic diseases. There are companies selling alkaline water or alkaline juices trying to ride this bandwagon. However, there isn't much scientific evidence to support these claims.

What is alkalinity? Alkalinity is the opposite of acidity. The water that we drink is neutral, hence it is tasteless. Anything acidic has a sour taste – that is why lemon, vinegar etc. taste sour. Alkaline stuff on the other hand tastes bitter. When something tastes bitter, it is an indication that our body does not want us to consume that stuff. It is an evolutionary programming.

The logic that is offered in support of alkaline stuff is that it reduces the acidity of the blood. More acidic blood is supposed to give rise to various diseases.

The reality is that the body maintains the pH (a measure of acidity/alkalinity) of our blood in a very tight range, because any large disturbance in it can be fatal. The balance is maintained by our lungs and kidneys. The lungs remove carbon dioxide (which is mildly acidic) from the blood, thus pushing it towards the alkaline side. This is an immediate action. For example, when you exercise, you produce more carbon dioxide, so you breathe faster to prevent the blood from becoming too acidic. The kidneys can reduce the acidity of the blood by excreting acids in urine. They also produce and regulate bicarbonate, which keeps the blood acidity in check. These actions take more time than those by the lungs and may take hours or days. This is how blood pH is maintained on short-term and long-term basis by the body.

Thus, our body is already well equipped to reduce the acidity of the blood and does not need outside help. And if the lungs and kidneys are not doing their job, then it is an emergency that requires immediate outside help – that of a hospital!

The acidity of the blood cannot be changed by drinking/eating alkaline stuff anyway, because this alkalinity cannot survive beyond the acid in our stomach. It is immediately neutralised in the stomach so cannot have any impact on the body beyond this point! Someone may argue that this reduces the acidity in the stomach, but the stomach acid is too strong to be dented by the slightly alkaline stuff you consume.

This whole story started when an animal study showed that alkaline water improved the health of some lab rats. It is not difficult to understand why... Water is made alkaline by dissolving minerals like calcium, potassium, magnesium, or iron. The lab rats are on a restricted diet so might have benefited from this extra dose of minerals.

In our case, we are already getting all these minerals through our food. Excess of these can be harmful. The human body has evolved to take good care of itself. The less we interfere with its functioning, the better...!

32.

Blue light from screens is bad...

Only at night!

There is a lot of hue and cry these days about the blue light from computer/mobile phone screens. A number of products, from screen filters to spectacle lenses to software that automatically changes the screen brightness are on the market to encash these blues against the blue light.

Blue light mimics natural daylight for the eyes. Therefore, the eyes send a signal to the brain that it is daytime. When this signal stops, the brain knows it is night-time. This triggers the release of a hormone called melatonin from the pineal gland in the brain. Melatonin prepares the body and brain to go to sleep. It also regulates the rhythms of the metabolism and other bodily functions to keep them in sync with our sleep-wake cycle.

If our eyes continue to receive the blue light long after the sunset, then the melatonin release is blocked because the brain is still getting the 'day time' signal. This disrupts the sleep-wake cycle and all the associated biological rhythms.

This disturbance has been linked to many chronic diseases. In addition, melatonin itself has antioxidant and anti-ageing properties. Decreased level of melatonin has been associated with increased risk of cancer. Women working in nightshifts have been found to have 50% higher risk of breast cancer.

When you continue to be exposed to blue light emitting sources late into the night, the melatonin secretion may remain blocked. This is the reason to avoid the practice entirely (ideally) and if you cannot, then it is advisable to use a blue light filter (hardware or software) during the night.

Some have taken it too far and insist on using such filters all the time, as if blue light is a poison for the eyes! Some companies selling spectacle lenses are offering lenses with permanent blue light filters. This is not advisable because we need both – the 'off' signal as well as the 'on' signal in equal measure to maintain the rhythm of our sleep-wake cycle. So, we don't want the blue light during the nighttime, but it is a good thing during the daytime so that the brain continues to receive the daytime signal, else it will disrupt the natural rhythm.

Many falsely believe that it is this blue light from screens that makes kids myopic (needing glasses for far sight). Earlier generations of parents believed that too much reading or watching TV made the eyes go weak.

Now scientific research has finally shown that not getting sufficient exposure to sunlight in early childhood distorts the eyeballs and causes myopia.

In closed spaces where you don't receive natural daylight, the blue light from your devices is actually a desirable daytime signal for your brain…!

33.

Tea is bad...

Think again!

Apart from the language in which this book is written, there are many things that came to India from the West and are now an inseparable part of our lives: potato, tomato, red chillies, rajma, coffee and tea!

Ever wondered how Indians entertained their guests before the arrival of tea/coffee? Well, India had a tradition of herbal teas made out of spices, herbs and milk. Now some organisations like ISKCON are trying to revive this tradition. In some communities, they used to offer opium water as a treat to their guests – this tradition of course is not worth reviving!

We have had a love-hate relationship with tea. Kids were threatened with 'dark complexion' when they asked for it. There is certainly no scientific evidence linking tea drinking to darkening of skin. Now many of these kids have grown up and have switched to coffee, seeing tea drinkers as old-fashioned.

Many still see drinking tea as something to be minimised as it causes 'acidity'. This is not entirely wrong as tea contains something known as 'tannin' that irritate the food pipe and the valve that separates the food pipe from the stomach. But these tannins can be tamed by adding a little protein to the tea – tannins bind to protein and will no longer be available to irritate your organs. Therefore, it is advisable to add milk. Even honey or lemon contain some protein and can do the job. Same is true for coffee. Boiling in water followed by boiling with sufficient milk does an even better job of binding the tannins. The 'dry mouth' feeling that you get after drinking black tea or black coffee is due to these tannins. The unbound tannins can also stain your teeth and teacups. Tannins can also leach out aluminium from a utensil and cause even more acidity, therefore never make tea in an aluminium pot.

In fact, tannins and caffeine are the two main constituents of tea and coffee. Caffeine has a stimulating effect, thus increasing the breathing rate and heart rate, mental alertness and physical energy. On the heart, it therefore has the same effect as exercise. Together these effects product a kind of refreshing feeling. So, caffeine is what we want; tannin is the price we pay for getting some caffeine!

In addition, both tea and coffee contain many compounds that have antioxidant and other beneficial properties. Tea has more of these and less of caffeine. Coffee has less of these and more of caffeine. These compounds have been linked to various health benefits such as improved blood circulation, reduced inflammation, lower risk of heart disease, cancer, piles, stroke, dementia etc. Research has shown a 1.5% lower risk of death from all causes for every cup of tea consumed daily. This should be the real reason to drink tea!

However, these compounds can also inhibit iron absorption from food, so tea/coffee should not be taken with food as a routine.

Tea also contains a substance called L-theanine, which can improve focus. L-theanine increases alpha activity in the brain, resulting in relaxation and better focus. This could be the reason behind individuals reporting more stable energy after drinking tea, compared to coffee or other caffeinated beverages. In this hypercompetitive world, you can't overstate the importance of focus, can you...?

Epilogue

The Times of India was running a campaign against fake news, with the slogan 'fake news has real consequences' at the time of writing this book. Every day, they showed examples of real individuals from different walks of life who had been harmed by fake news.

I was writing on almost the same subject, but it's an irony that the victims of the kind of fake news I have written against are a faceless multitude. Because when someone is robbed of money, they run to the police. But when someone is robbed of health, they don't even know what happened!

Edward Wilson said, 'We have stone-age emotions, medieval institutions and god-like technology'. The god-like technology is misused to take us for a ride, our stone-age emotions are easily fooled, and our medieval institutions are clueless as to what to do about it!

So, someone has to do something about it. As Alan Turing said, 'We can only see a short distance ahead, but we can see plenty there that needs to be done'.

Therefore, I have included in this book whatever I could see. There could be a lot more out there. What we need is to develop an attitude against believing and acting on the same, and an aptitude for doing our own research and fact-checking.

During Covid there was rampant disinformation going around against the Covid vaccine, that it will cause cancer, or one will die within so many days etc. Some poor souls ran away from cities and hid in their villages to avoid vaccination. The West is fighting its own battle against the so called anti-vaxxers, who refuse vaccination and link it with autism and what not.

Then there are the cancer-classics like biopsy needles spread cancer and that microwave ovens cause cancer and the latest one that 5G technology will cause cancer.

Issues during Covid brought the problem of digital disinformation to the centre stage, and now even the UN is getting involved. António Guterres, United Nations Secretary-General says "Countering disinformation requires lasting investment in building societal resilience and media and information literacy" while trying to promote international cooperation in countering disinformation.

While 'investment in building media and information literacy' is something that is best done by governments and enterprises, 'building societal resilience' is what individuals can contribute to, through whatever means of communication we can find.

Print media is one such means as it can cut through the digital clutter. That was the idea behind this book.

So spread the truth around and stay safe!

Acknowledgements for graphs/diagrams:

Effects on blood glucose over time:
https://www.dietdoctor.com/blood-sugar

Blood sugar level, glucose vs. apple:
https://www.baliza.de/en/article/glycemic-index-load.html

Blood sugar profile, with and without activity:
https://novi-health.com/education/walking-after-meals-l8rtj

Blood sugar and age:
https://www.research.colostate.edu/healthyagingcenter/aging-basics/blood-sugar/

Basal metabolic rate and age: http://www.fitnesshealth101.com/index.php?option=com_content&view=article&id=22&Itemid=33

24-hour energy expenditure vs. muscle mass:
https://blogs.brighton.ac.uk/obesitygroup2974/strength-training/